LIGHTEN UP YOUR BODY,
LIGHTEN UP YOUR LIFE

BOOKS BY LUCIA CAPACCHIONE

The Power of Your Other Hand: A Course in Channeling the Inner Wisdom of the Right Brain. Newcastle Publishing Co., Inc.

The Creative Journal: The Art of Finding Yourself. Newcastle Publishing Co., Inc.

The Well-Being Journal: Drawing on Your Inner Power to Heal Yourself. Newcastle Publishing Co., Inc.

Lighten Up Your Body, Lighten Up Your Life (Co-authored with James Strohecker and Elizabeth Johnson). Newcastle Publishing Co., Inc.

The Creative Journal for Children: A Guide for Parents, Teachers and Counselors
The Picture of Health: Healing Your Life with Art. Hay House, Inc.
Recovery of Your Inner Child. Simon & Schuster
Audio Tape *The Picture of Health & Healing Your Life With Art.* Hay House, Inc.

For information regarding LUCIA CAPACCHIONE's books, lectures, workshops, and consultations contact:
LUCIA CAPACCHIONE
P.O. Box 5805
Santa Monica, CA 90409
(213) 281-7495

LIGHTEN UP YOUR BODY, LIGHTEN UP YOUR LIFE

Beyond Diet & Exercise: The
Inner Path to Lasting Change

LUCIA CAPACCHIONE, Ph.D.
ELIZABETH JOHNSON, M.A.
JAMES STROHECKER

NEWCASTLE PUBLISHING CO., INC.
NORTH HOLLYWOOD, CALIFORNIA
1990

ISBN 0-87877-150-6

Edited by Nancy Shaw Strohecker
Cover Design by Riley K. Smith

The authors of this book do not dispense medical advice nor prescribe the
use of any technique as a form of treatment for medical problems without
the advice of a physician, either directly or indirectly. The intent of the authors
is only to offer information of a general nature to help you cooperate with
your doctor in your mutual quest for health. In the event you use any of the
information in this book for yourself, you are prescribing for yourself, which
is your constitutional right, but the authors and publishers assume no responsibility for your actions.

A NEWCASTLE BOOK
First printing, February 1990
10 9 8 7 6 5
Printed in the United States of America

Dedicated

To The "Light Body" Living Within You

THANKS

to the contributors:

Donna Jean Barnard
Lucia Capacchione
Terri Freas
Nancy Graham
Elizabeth Johnson
Ann Parenti
Tom Stitzel
James Strohecker
Marge Windisch

Contents

Foreword

I discovered the work of Lucia Capacchione in 1985. I had just moved to California having left New York and my fitness business of twenty years. I was looking for a new way to experience and work with my body, as I had found the old way didn't work for me anymore. I was in the Bodhi Tree Bookstore in Los Angeles, and came across a spiral-bound book called *Lighten Up Journal: Making Friends With Your Body*, by Lucia Capacchione and Elizabeth Johnson. It was a workbook for getting in touch with one's body, weight issues, and image. And, although I am a leader in the field of fitness and body awareness, getting in touch with my own body was a new experience. This workbook was one of the great tools which helped me create the body I wanted, while making peace with my body.

You are married to your body. It is with you morning, noon, and night during every change in season, through sickness and health. You wake up with it, go to sleep with it, and always find your self right where you left off, in the body you were born with. The body is your vehicle in life, and the physical manifestation of your thoughts and beliefs. It is what your soul has specially chosen for you to learn your particular lessons in this life. And it is time to make peace with it, to love it, and to know that you and it are perfect just the way you are in your life now.

For so many of us, the body we live in does not measure up to what we think we "should" have. It does not look "picture perfect," and a battle of self against self takes place throughout life. No matter how hard one tries to deny it, and no matter how strange it may seem, loving your body is the key to having the body you want. Loving yourself is the key for creating a high quality of life.

The book you have in your hands will help you to do just that. It is an exquisite journey of self-discovery, joy, and self-love. In *Lighten Up Your*

Body, Lighten Up Your Life, you now have an opportunity to discover new ways of communicating with yourself. You will discover beliefs that have held you back or kept you "stuck." You will learn to release the beliefs that no longer work for you, "unstick" yourself, and move into a more joyous way of being. You will do this through writing, drawing, and journal work.

Lucia Capacchione, the creator of this method, is a personal friend and guide for me. A remarkable woman with a remarkable gift, she teaches you how to "feel" your body; something you may have forgotten how to do. And as you begin to remember, all the good feelings you ever had begin to return. You will rediscover how very special your own feelings are. And with this knowledge comes the understanding of how magnificent your body is. You will get to re-experience the joy of your own uniqueness, and the special way in which only you can express and create the kind of body and life you want. In this wonderful process, you can recreate a relationship with yourself and become your own best friend. And unlike any other friendship, this one will be with you every moment for the rest of your life.

You are now embarking on one of the most exciting of adventures; the adventure of your Self. I wish you all the joy, happiness, inner peace and self-love that you will find at the end of this journey. But the end of this adventure is merely the beginning of the greatest of all adventures; your new life in your new body. Have fun, dear reader, you are a special being filled with light and wisdom—after all, you picked up this book.

Congratulations.

> With love and light,
> and peels of laughter,
>
> Suzy Prudden
> Creator of:
> *MetaFitness®, Your Thoughts Taking Shape*

Preface

This book is intended as a guide and road map for the inner journey to reclaim your true body, and experience it as your friend. It contains a series of activities, each with its own descriptive title, theme, and purpose. You may want to read the entire book through once to familiarize yourself with the process. Or you may be inspired to do the activities right away. In either case, in order to benefit from this book you will need to experience it and do it for yourself.

After you are familiar with the activities, use the book in any sequence or manner you wish. Find the activity that best suits your needs. Let your inner voice lead you to the appropriate technique for exploring whatever personal issue you are dealing with at the time. Above all, set aside your self-criticism and be creative. Make these exercises your own, and see the amazing results in your body and your self-image!

LIGHT AND **HEAVY**

Light	**Heavy**
Happy	**Depressed**
Transparent	**Gloomy**
Cheerful	**Bulky**
Carefree	**Dense**
Levity	**Sad**
Light-hearted	**Heavy-hearted**
Graceful	**Burdened**
Fluid	**Weighty**
Thin	**Massive**
Lightweight	**Heavyweight**
Enlightened	**Clumsy**
Flowing	**Somber**
Revealed	**Heavy-set**
Effortless	**Gravity**
Delicate	**Serious**
Radiance	**Grave**
Bright	**Oppressive**
Illuminated	**Cumbersome**
Joyous	**Ponderous**

CHAPTER ONE

From the Inside Out

We shall not cease from exploration
And the end of all our exploring
Will be to arrive where we started
And know the place for the first time.

—T. S. Eliot

You are about to begin a wonderful jouney. The goal of this journey is a simple one—to discover the body that nature intended for you. This body feels "light," unencumbered, and is a joy to live in. It not only feels light, but it looks light and vibrant to the eye. And it radiates a glow of vitality and health. Does all this sound impossible to you? If so, you are in for a big surprise. The good news is that this body already lives within you right now. We call it your "Light Body."

Your Light Body is not created or put on from the outside. It is not attained through cosmetic surgery, deprivation and crash diets, weekend weight reduction programs, or compulsive exercise. To the contrary, your Light Body emerges as a natural result of a healthy and balanced life. This book will help you liberate your true Light Body.

You will know you have arrived at your destination *when you feel at home in your body.* Your Light Body has nothing to do with how much you weigh or what size clothing you wear. Furthermore, it can never be measured by ideal or stereotypical forms seen in magazines, television shows, and movies. In fact, your Light Body is not defined by physical appearance. It is not determined by others on the outside looking in. Your Light Body is experienced from the *inside looking out*—a feeling of being comfortable in your own body. However, when you discover your Light Body, *you will look and feel different*—to yourself and others.

1

Our body is an intelligent and perfectly designed work of nature fully capable of regulating and healing itself. Nature did not intend for us to live our lives feeling sluggish, heavy, burdened, and at odds with our bodies. We were meant to feel "light" in our bodies. However, over the years many of us have buried our Light Bodies under layers of repressed emotions, limiting beliefs, and negative attitudes about ourselves and our bodies.

In this day and age, we are fed a steady diet of advertising images and impossible standards to live up to, epitomized by the popular saying, "You can't be too rich or too thin." We are a nation obsessed with status and appearances. Our standards of beauty and attractiveness have spawned enormous industries—fitness, weight control, health and beauty care, and cosmetic surgery—which cater to the unrelenting perfectionist in us all. How can our bodies possibly thrive when we are constantly scrutinizing them, and trying to make them into objects—something they are not? Once you buy into the abstract notion of the *ideal* body, the "perfect 10," you have fallen into a downward spiral that only breeds dissatisfaction and unhealthy competition with others. Many people spend thousands of dollars on fitness and exercise classes, expensive sports gear, diet plans, and cosmetic surgery, all in a desperate attempt to obtain the elusive "perfect" body. Even if they capture it for a time, the price they pay is very stiff. And without constant vigilance the "image" mysteriously disappears.

On the other hand, there are those who give up in a state of despair and hopelessness. Aliens in their own bodies, they reconcile themselves to failure and a chronic dissatisfaction with their body image. Others continue to vacillate between the two extremes: lose and gain, lose and gain. Bursts of fitness activity are followed by "failure" and futility. Does this relentless cycle sound familiar?

The fact is, however, that outer change not accompanied by *inner change* will never last. Like a rubber band the body can only snap back to its old shape because it is molded by our unconscious belief system and emotional patterns. LIGHTENING UP, FEELING AT HOME IN YOUR BODY, IS A PROCESS WHICH CAN ONLY HAPPEN FROM THE INSIDE OUT. This process includes all of you: your feelings, thoughts, beliefs, and lifestyle.

In workshops we often ask if anyone is happy with their body and physical appearance. It is very rare for anyone to give an unequivocal, "yes." In fact, it is our experience that the very people who are held up as "ideal" models of physical beauty are no happier with their bodies than anyone else.

One thing becomes very clear: If we have low self-esteem we will not feel good about our bodies, regardless of how we appear to the world. The reverse is true as well; not liking our body is a great excuse for not liking ourselves. We can always find things about our bodies that do not "measure up" to society's standards as we perceive them.

This raises the whole issue of motivation. Why do we want to change? Is it to please others and gain their approval? Is it to "earn" love? Is it to feel powerful because we look good, and are able to attract and/or reject others? In this book we will explore the question: "Who are you doing this for?" And we will show you how to grow into the healthy and balanced attitude, "I am doing it for me."

LUCIA'S STORY

When I was a child I longed to be a dancer. I grew up with film images of great stars like Fred Astaire, Ginger Rogers, Gene Kelly, Cyd Charisse, and Leslie Caron. My father, a film editor at MGM studios, worked on many of the great musicals of the forties. And my mother used to take me to the ballet, live on a stage! I was enthralled with the dazzling sets and costumes and, of course, the dancing.

However, after being diagnosed with a minor heart murmur when I was quite young, my well-meaning but overprotective mother would not allow me to take dance lessons. My heart was broken when my best friend went off to ballet class. I wanted so much to wear a tutu and satin toe-shoes. Secretly, I used to dance around my room trying to stand on my toes. However, I felt frustrated and angry because I wanted to study dance. But expressions of anger were not acceptable in our household, so my only way out of this dilemma was to unconsciously deaden those emotions. I did this by overeating, which *was* acceptable in my family and in our Italian sub-culture.

I grew up with a body image which was programmed into my mind by my family and peers. "I am chubby, awkward, and clumsy. I'm not athletic and would make a fool of myself if I tried playing competitive sports such as volleyball or basketball. If I overexert myself I'll get sick (and maybe die)." To make matters worse, during the years that I was forming this belief system, my favorite uncle and my grandmother died. At this time my father had a very serious case of pneumonia. My mother's injunction "Don't run around too much, you'll catch your death of pneumonia," struck fear in my heart. Unfortunately, like a dutiful daughter I fulfilled her prophecy, and came down with a serious case of pneumonia when I was nine years old, thereby proving that "Mother was right."

From that time on until college, I struggled with weight. I can remember being taken to a doctor and put on a diet plan at fourteen years of age. It was a nightmare because the underlying emotional cause of my overeating was never addressed. Like all such one-dimensional approaches to weight loss, this one was a miserable failure. It added layers of shame and guilt to an already damaged body image.

On top of everything else, I was struggling with the usual dilemmas of adolescence in a *highly unusual* setting: Hollywood. Many of my classmates at Immaculate Heart High School were daughters of movie industry celebrities, or girls being groomed for careers in film, television, and theater. One girl left school in order to accept a role in a hit Broadway musical, another was modeling hair fashions in national magazines, and another classmate went on to become a film and television star. The models of "perfection" which most people see only in magazines and on the screen, sat across the aisle from me in the classroom. Comparing myself to such a standard of beauty while going through the awkward teenage years was very depressing, to say the least.

College was my salvation. The glamour girls had all gone into the entertainment industry, and I was now surrounded with young women like myself. We loved books and learning, and we thrived on creative expression through art. My heroine was my teacher, the well-known artist, Sister Mary Corita. She was decidedly not a glamour girl. She recognized that I had both creative ability and a commitment to art. What I looked like or what I wore did not matter to her. She cared about what I expressed. I blossomed and soared. I lost weight almost immediately after entering college—a time when most young women start putting on weight—without diet, exercise, or any other effort. The secret was that I was happy and doing what I loved most: painting, drawing, designing sets, acting in plays, going to parties and DANCING into the early hours. I was in my element, and my body image changed dramatically reflecting my joyful and creative state.

For the first time since early childhood I enjoyed living in my body. I had my own car and did as I pleased. I stopped fighting the battle with my body and became my own person. I finally felt and looked attractive. After years of wearing uniforms in Catholic elementary and high schools, I discovered the art of dressing creatively. Combining ethnic jewelry and fabrics in unusual color combinations became a new medium of expression, a wonderful way to celebrate the new feelings about my body. I truly felt like a multi-colored butterfly that had emerged from a drab, dark cocoon.

After graduating from college, I married and became the mother of two young children who were fifteen months apart. I had lost much of the physical freedom and enjoyment I had experienced during college and my early twenties. I now felt "weighted down" by the serious responsibilities of family, and work as an artist and teacher. Unable to shed the extra pounds gained during pregnancy, I tried everything from diet pills to liquid diets. For the next few years I watched my weight go up and down.

The problem accelerated as I took on more career challenges. In the wake of the Watts riots in 1965, I was appointed to direct twelve Head Start pre-school centers located throughout Los Angeles County. I loved the job of training and supervising teachers in such a worthwhile program, but the work was extremely stressful. The commute was long, the work hours even longer, and of course I had family responsibilities waiting for me at home. With such an exhausting schedule, the only way I knew to nurture myself was to eat. Soon I weighed as much as I had when I was fourteen years old.

In looking back, I feel there was another reason for the weight gain. I was twenty-eight years old when I became a Head Start supervisor and I looked much younger than my age. Most of the other supervisors in the County were much older than I, and they did not take me seriously because of my youthful appearance. Our program had an excellent reputation, but when I was introduced to other supervisors at meetings many of them refused to accept me as a peer. They would say things like, "But you can't *possibly* be a supervisor. You're too young." Unconsciously, I felt that I needed to "carry more weight" (as in having more authority), so I gained extra pounds and felt "older." I looked and acted as if I were middle-aged. Many years later, both my daughters told me that during these years they thought I was actually in my forties.

After two years as a supervisor, I completely burned out and resigned from my position. I did, however, stay on as a part-time consultant, allowing me the time and freedom to pursue what I loved most, the creative arts. I began doing freelance design and film work in the beautiful, semi-rural environment of my home. Thus, I was no longer commuting and putting in long work hours at the office. With a less stressful lifestyle, the extra weight dropped off instantly and without effort.

The next few years were extremely challenging, including a divorce, minor illnesses, and many changes of residence. During this time, I found myself on the weight gain/weight loss see-saw again, and tried every diet and exercise program I could find. Ironically, it was not until I faced a life-threatening illness that I began to consciously heal my relationship with my body "from the inside out." I did this through personal journal work, therapy, acupressure, and bodywork. After years of struggling with weight fluctuation, I finally got off the roller coaster when I uncovered my buried feelings: anger, frustration, loneliness, grief, and fear. At thirty-eight years of age, I changed careers and became an art therapist, applying my experience and knowledge of the healing power of creative expression. I also uprooted destructive beliefs and planted new, life-giving ones, and my body lightened up and reshaped itself. At thirty-nine I took my first dance class, and within a year I performed in a community dance ensemble: a dream come true.

As an art therapist, I have shared my personal experiences in my battle with weight and body image with hundreds of students and clients. In offering the same techniques which helped me make peace with my own body, I have seen many people transform their bodies and their lives. One such person is my good friend and a co-author of this book, Elizabeth Johnson.

ELIZABETH'S STORY

One day, when I was thirty-one years old, I realized I was fat. Now, that may sound a little strange, but it is true. It was as if fat-filled-flesh had simply grown on me overnight. Suddenly, I realized that none of my clothes really fit very well and I could not even zip up my most beloved pair of jeans. On my way to work, wearing a loose-fitting frock and sandals, I wondered, "How had this happened?"

It's a funny thing about "wondering." We can "wonder" forever without taking any action—which is just about what I did. I "wondered" why I gained so much weight while I kept getting fatter and fatter. After a year or so I decided, rather half-heartedly, to try to do something about this extra baggage carried on my bones. So began the long succession of diets.

I say "half-heartedly," because by this time I was feeling very unhappy about my appearance, and my self-esteem was so low that I had rejected all the things that had always brought me joy: clothes, shopping, interior design, walks in the hills, sports, visiting new places, being at the beach, creative writing, even sex. However, I did not give up music. I would listen to music for hours in the safety and privacy of my own home. Once in a while, though, I would try to move to the music, and would feel so stupid that I would immediately give up. I never felt so fat and embarrassed of myself.

For several years the succession of diets was an on-going, non-stop adventure in boredom and disappointment. I tried every diet that I could get my hands on in a large metropolitan city. That is a lot. I even made up my own diet—sandwiches wrapped in lettuce instead of bread. This was truly an experiement in personal deprivation!

On the off-handed suggestion of a friend, which had nothing to do with the topic of weight, I enrolled in *Creative Journal* weekend classes at a local community college, conducted by Lucia Capacchione. The workshops were wonderful, and I began studying more and more the concepts and techniques that Lucia had originated with her *Creative Journal* method. I, quite happily, became a "journal junkie."

Time passed and although I had addressed the issue of my extra weight many times in my own journals, nothing seemed to change on the outside of me. However, the "inner me" was jumping and leaping with new awarenesses. Through journal activities I came to realize that, for quite some time prior to my weight gain, my dear little self had been under tremendous stress: my father had died; I had been through two beautiful/devastating relationships; and a young friend passed away. Also, many years spent in the music business had brought hectic travel, low pay, little appreciation, and very little joy. I had been feeling wounded for a long, long time. People do various things to prevent themselves from being hurt. I protected myself with a lot of extra weight.

Then something happened—something both subtle and dynamic. One Saturday morning in early January, I somehow caught a glimpse of my upper back and shoulders in the dresser mirror. "Oh dear," I thought, "really elderly women have nicer backs than this." I remember that instant as though it happened this morning. I then put on baggy sweats, drove to the local dance studio, and took my first aerobics class. I knew no one in class and had little idea of exactly what they were doing, but I left that class feeling that I was really breathing for the first time in many years. When I got home I spent the rest of the afternoon reviewing my old journals. Guess what I found?

Whenever I had done an activity on how to get rid of the extra weight, I had always told myself the same thing: eat salads and dance. For over two years of journal-keeping, the same information on my weight control was revealed to me: eat salads and dance. It could have been a left/right hand dialogue, a drawing, a conversation, a squiggle, the information was the same: eat salads and dance. I HAD NOT LISTENED! I, quite simply, had not listened to what I was telling myself to do.

Now I listened and acted upon the information. By April I had "lost," "released," "gotten rid of," "given up," thirty pounds. Exercise and salads were now a very natural part of my life. In September I very tentatively took my first jazz class. One year later, I was performing modern and jazz dance on stage, in front of audiences. Me! Me, in costume and quite happy, performing to wonderful music in front of people! It had not been all that long ago that I sat in my living room listening to music, feeling too fat and unhappy to move.

There is more. In 1989 I decided to leave Los Angeles and relocate in New England. All plans were going very smoothly, and guess what? I noticed that a couple of my dresses were getting a little snug, and I realized that I had been skipping quite a few dance classes. This time, without hesitation, I listened to myself in my journal. My Inner Child was scared and she wanted protection. So I protected myself-as-my-child by taking long walks with the dog (dog = protection), making sure I had enough money to make this move (money = protection). I also researched the area and called ahead to establish business relationships (knowledge = protection). For me, extra weight does not equal protection anymore. My suggestion is that we all LISTEN to the advice and suggestions revealed in our journals, and then act on it.

> *Whatever you think or believe you can do, begin it.*
> *For in action, there is magic, grace, and power.*
>
> —Goethe

JAMES' STORY

I enjoyed an unusual childhood, growing up in a "secret city" tucked away in the green, rolling hills of East Tennessee. Constructed during World War II by the govenment as part of the Manhattan Project, Oak Ridge was surrounded by natural beauty. The rivers, lakes, mountains, and endless forests made it a veritable childhood paradise. It also offered a flourishing intellectual and cultural environment, fostered by the challenges of the newly born Atomic age and the utopian vision of the city's founders. In fact, as children we were led to believe that we had the finest educational system in the country, and there was an unspoken belief that we were somehow "different" and "special." Because of this attitude, both the pressures to excel and the standards of excellence were very high.

My hometown also developed a strong athletic tradition, and sports were a great source of civic pride. However, as a young boy sports were a challenge due to my size. I was often teased for being all skin and bones. Not only was I very skinny, I was also short. In fact, my family nicknames were "shorty" and "shrimp." As the youngest of three children, I remember being constantly surrounded by "bigger" people in my early childhood and feeling "small" and somehow unimportant. The fact that I was considered "cute" was not very reassuring.

I grew up in the fifties and sixties when the "he-man" ideal body image was popular. I will never forget all the magazine ads for the muscle-man, Charles Atlas, showing a "98 pound weakling" getting sand kicked in his face at the beach by a mean, over-sized bully. Although I felt these ads were ridiculous, they still subconsciously reinforced the belief that gaining a "Mr. America" physique was the best way to get rid of the bullies and get all the girls. This belief was further reinforced by the childhood rituals of arm-wrestling, hand-squeezing, slugging, and making "muscles." Slowly I succumbed to a modern American myth.

In grade school, I began looking for ways to "beef up" my muscles and get stronger. My motivation was strengthened by the desire to emulate my older brother who was much bigger and more muscular than I was. At this time I developed two beliefs: "Exercising and lifting weights will give me the body I desire," and "If I eat enough I will become big and strong." I ate like a horse (to my mother's dismay, I am sure), and lifted weights religiously. My best friend and I weighed ourselves almost daily, and measured our height, chests, necks, waists, biceps, thighs, and calves. Although thin, I was very athletic and constantly played baseball, football, basketball, and tennis. I ran, jumped, tumbled, and even tried boxing. As I watched my strength increase with all these activities, the size and shape of my body changed very little.

During junior high I matured at a rate much slower than the boys my age, and I also had two operations on my knee to remove a cyst. My body now seemed to be unpredictable and unreliable, and for the first time in my life I began to distrust it. To compound matters, I was only 5'3" tall at the age of thirteen. My height seemed to work against me. In eighth grade I was cut from the junior varsity basketball team, although I was more skilled than some of the tall, gawky players who were kept only for their height.

I was a late bloomer, however. Suddenly, at fifteen my body began to shoot up like a tree, and by the time I was a senior in high school, I had grown to 6'3" and 190 pounds. Overnight, I was "big" and people began to react to me in a different manner. My experience was something like the child in the movie *Big*, who woke up one morning in an adult body after wishing that he were big. In two years I went from playing a short guard to a tall center on my basketball team. The football coach wondered where I had been hiding the year before. I earned a whole new set of family nicknames, such as "giant," "monster," and "the tree." However, it took a few years for the "shorty" self-image to wear off, and for me to feel at home in my new body.

Still, I believed that I needed to have that chiseled, "Mr. America" body. On weekends, I would sneak through the window of my High School gym to use all of the special weight equipment. I did isometric exercises, ran, jumped rope, tried to eat healthy foods, and really focused on developing my physique. I learned how to lift weights not only with physical strength, but through directing energy with my mind. However, with all the sports and physical activities, nothing seemed to really make me happy and content. I was very self-critical and began believing that we were not really meant to be at peace with our bodies.

Then during my senior year in college, I had a very unusual experience that forever transformed the way I looked and felt about my body. I was sitting in the bathtub just gazing at my body. Suddenly, my entire body was bathed in a beautiful, soft golden light. It seemed so perfect and magnificent despite its "imperfections." For the first time in my life, I really felt at home in my body. At that moment, I began to truly love and honor my body, not because of its appearance, but because I experienced it as a sacred gift. It seemed to be a holy temple which contained a valuable, mysterious treasure.

Shortly after this experience I met Mary Candler Smith, a remarkable woman in her late sixties who had lived in India for nearly twenty-five years, and now lived close to my home in Oak Ridge. I began studying hatha yoga and meditation with her and immediately noticed dramatic changes in how I felt and looked. Although I was somewhat slimmer, I was stronger and more balanced. My body began to feel light and fluid, and I seemed to glide effortlessly through my daily activities. Often, while practicing yoga I would experience my body as pure, radiant energy. During these times I would gradually lose the sense of "having" a physical body. Instead, I began to live *in and through* my body.

I continued studying yoga and meditation for several years in India with the late spiritual master, Swami Muktananda. Through meditation my experience of the body as a form of energy continued to deepen. It became clear that we are much more than blood, flesh, and bones—every atom of our gross, physical body is permeated with consciousness and energy. I learned to love and honor the body as a temple for this conscious energy—the Inner Self.

A few years later I was in a serious automobile accident in which my car was totalled by two trucks, and my body absorbed a great deal of shock. I began to experience pain, numbness, and problems with motor coordination. I no longer experienced being light, fluid, and "at home" in my body. In fact, it was very unpleasant and uncomfortable to be in my body. Due to this condition, I was unable to exercise or practice hatha yoga. Thus began a lifelong quest to relieve my discomfort and restore the sense of lightness and balance which I had lost. I explored acupuncture, acupressure, chiropractic, physical therapy, herbs, imagery, stress reduction, cranioscral therapy, massage, and structural bodywork. I also experienced many forms of movement work and body awareness, including the Feldenkrais Method, the Alexander Technique, Aston Patterning, and Embodiment.

Through all of this exploration I received no lasting relief, so I decided to take matters into my own hands. I began to study various forms of movement awareness, bodywork, and imagery in order to learn how to take care of myself. My greatest teacher, however, was my own body. It taught me how to heal from the inside out. Slowly, I began to rediscover a sense of lightness and energy, primarily through the regenerating effects of deep relaxation. Although I was unable to execute yoga postures, I was able to practice rhythmic yogic breathing. This allowed me to descend into deeper and deeper states of relaxation, in which I experienced a tangible shift in my bodily awareness. My body no longer seemed solid or physical. Instead, I experienced it as a field of energy, just as I had during my earlier practice of yoga. In this state, I also observed that the body's innate intelligence and self-regulating powers were free to operate with little or no resistance, helping to bring about healing and regeneration. Often, my "inner physician" would naturally and spontaneously bring about the same physical changes in my muscles, connective tissue, and structural alignment that I wold normally experience after an hour session of movement or bodywork.

While on my own healing journey, I began sharing my knowledge and experience with others. I developed an approach to helping people in re-connecting with their bodies and themselves, which I call *Body/Mind Balance*. My work focuses on the direct experience of the Light Body through relaxation, breathing, gentle bodywork and movement, and giving tools to reinforce that experience in everyday life. From my work, I have learned that when we look at our bodies we normally focus on our outer shell or armoring, and are unaware of the Light Body concealed within. Naturally, we feel dissatisfied. On the other hand, when we experience our Light Body, not only do we look good to others, we look good to *ourselves* as well. In order to reveal this hidden treasure, however, it is necessary to do some inner work and to examine and change old, limiting beliefs and behavior patterns. The resulting emergence of our Light Body greatly enhances the process of embodying and living our own truth.

SELF-DISCOVERY THROUGH ART

Many of the activities in this book invite you to draw or create collages with pictures from magazines. Initially, you may resist this idea with the excuse that "you don't have any talent." Our experience shows that anyone can draw if they will just give it a try. Both drawing and writing come from the same ability. Making marks on paper which symbolize or represent our experiences is an innate human characteristic. The only thing that prevents us from drawing is the belief that we cannot do it. This is a learned belief and it can be unlearned. Since the work you are doing in this book is private, and not subject to the criticism of others, this is a safe context in which to relax and enjoy drawing for your eyes only. You will not be asked to make representational drawings of the outside world. Rather, you will be expressing your inner world on paper, discovering yourself through art.

THE POWER OF YOUR OTHER HAND

A special writing technique which we will frequently use in this book is the right hand/left hand dialogue. Yes, that's right. You will be writing with both hands. First one, and then the other. In this way you will be shown how to converse with many aspects of your life, in order to gain understanding and receive guidance from within. This dialogue technique was developed over the last fifteen years in which thousands of individuals have used it to achieve major breakthroughs. The development and other applications of this technique are discussed in greater detail in Lucia's book, *The Power of Your Other Hand.*

Some of you may be ambidextrous, or do some things with your right hand and other things with your left hand. But when you are instructed to use your NON-DOMINANT HAND in this book, please use your non-writing hand. Writing and drawing with your non-dominant hand can be just as scary as being asked to do artwork. It will probably feel strange at first, but with practice and perseverance the results will far outweigh any awkwardness or embarrassment that you may experience. In writing with your non-dominant hand, do not worry about your spelling, grammar, or penmanship. If you can learn to accept sloppy handwriting, you will be able to reach an inner wisdom and truth that you have never known before.

CREATIVE JOURNAL-KEEPING

Keeping a personal journal is a powerful way to bring about change in your life. Most of the exercises in this book are designed to be done in a journal or notebook. If you already keep a diary or journal, you may want to expand and include these activities. If you have never kept a journal, that is fine. You will be given clear guidelines. However, this approach to journal-keeping is unique as it combines both drawing and writing. Through art you can draw upon deeper levels of your creative unconscious to discover your true feelings and to change beliefs which are not serving you. Through writing you can articulate and clarify your insights in order to apply them to everyday life. Once you begin keeping a "Lighten Up" journal, you may find it useful in all areas of your life.

The activities in this book complement medically supervised health care, nutrition and exercise programs, psychotherapy, bodywork, and support groups. Use it in conjunction with everything you are doing to improve your health and body image.

GUIDELINES

As you embark upon the exercises, here are some important guidelines to keep in mind:

1) PRIVACY — Keep your work in a private, safe place. Confidentiality is important as it will allow you to be honest and to express yourself freely without judgment from others. You may want to share certain passages or drawings with people you trust such as a counselor or friend. Be selective and avoid showing your work to people who tend to criticize or control you.

2) SETTING — When you are ready to do the exercises, find a quiet, comfortable place where you will not be interrupted or distracted. For some people this is difficult to do. If that is the case, then figuring out how to create privacy for yourself will be an important step in your own growth.

3) TIME — You do not have to do exercises from this book every day in order to benefit from them. Do the exercises when you choose. However, when you decide to work with the material, reserve a block of fifteen minutes of work time or more. Some of them may take longer so schedule your time appropriately. For optimal results we recommend

using these exercises a minimum of 3–4 times a week. However, feel absolutely free to use your journal whenever you wish. Date each entry and keep them in chronological order. This will be helpful when you look back over your work to see your progress. Some amazing discoveries have been made through this kind of review.

4) RELAXATION — Creativity flows more naturally when you are relaxed, so it is helpful to become as relaxed as possible before you begin work. Use a relaxation technique of your choice or simply sit with closed eyes and observe the rhythm of your breath. Chapter 2 contains a relaxation technique which you can use throughout the book.

5) MATERIALS — You will need the following materials:

A notebook with unlined white paper (8–1/2″ × 11″) such as the following:

> A three-ring binder,
> A spiral sketch pad, or
> A blank book (hardbound or paperback)

Unlined white paper (8–1/2″ × 11″ or larger)

Colored felt pens (assortment of eight or more colors)

Crayons

Oil or chalk pastels (optional)

Scissors and glue

Magazines with photographs such as *Life, Better Homes and Gardens, Vogue, GQ, Sports Illustrated, National Geographic, Lears, Architectural Digest.*

Enjoy the wonderful adventure before you in discovering your own Light Body!

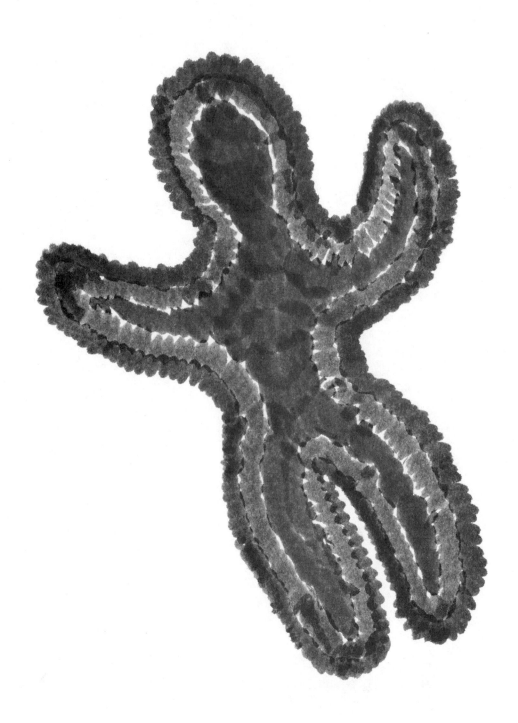

CHAPTER TWO

Making Friends With Your Body

One is one's own friend or one's own enemy.

—Bhagavad Gita

Lightening up the body starts with BEING IN the body. When we started out as infants, we were fully present in our bodies. However, early in life many of us learned to "split off" from our body in response to trauma, such as emotional or physical abuse. We attempted to escape the pain of these experiences by dissociating from our bodily sensations and going "into our heads." Instead of living in our bodies, we began to live in our thoughts, fantasies, and daydreams. We lost touch with our physical sensations, our gut instincts, our true feelings, and our wants and needs. The body became a battlefield. We listened to what others said we should want and feel, and stopped listening to our own selves.

This split may be rooted in early infancy for those of us who were raised during the era of "scheduled feedings." Our infant cries (signaling hunger) were ignored by clock-watching adults. Although the time-table approach was supposedly devised for the good of the infant, it was really based on adults needs for control and convenience. Fortunately, feeding upon demand (along with natural childbirth and breast-feeding) have come back into favor in the last twenty years. But we now have at least two generations of people who were affected by insensitive and unhealthy feeding methods. In dealing with issues of weight and self-image, it is essential to understand the roots of our disconnectedness from our bodies. If we learned from our caregivers that our own body's messages did not count, and that the decisions about how much we should eat were in the hands of others, we learned to devalue our body's true needs.

Cut off from our physical sensations, we were put at a severe disadvantage in determining our own needs.

Is it any wonder that many of us lost our self-esteem in this damaging process of being disconnected from our bodies? This situation inevitably leads to confusion and an emotional emptiness which calls out to be filled. The problem is that we do not know how to fill our emotional needs, so we compensate by overeating and abusing other substances. After the body has had enough, there is still a gnawing emptiness which is misunderstood as a call for food. Habitually overfeeding the body becomes a substitute for feeding the heart and soul.

When we "Lighten Up" we listen to the body, trust its messages, and respond with love and care. We respect the body's truth and create a lifestyle which honors our "bodyself." For regardless of what we do to raise our self-esteem, if we do not feel good about our bodies, then we are lost, homeless, and forced to search for something *outside* to make us feel good *inside*. Our own bodies are the first and last home we will have on this planet. They make us human and they also contain—in every cell—a deeper inner knowing by which we can guide ourselves to the light of truth.

In this first series of writing and drawing activities, you learn how to make friends with your body. Through drawings and dialogues you explore the body image which you hold in your mind. Thus, by learning to listen to what your body is saying, you take the first steps in "coming home" to yourself. As you become resensitized to physical sensations, you see how your body is shaped by the emotions held deep inside. After looking at your current body-image, you are invited to create the picture of your "Light" Body—the body which nature intended for you.

Revere the body and care for it, for it is a temple.

—Swami Muktananda

HOW I SEE MY BODY

Sit comfortably with your journal or notebook and colored felt pens. Close your eyes and take a moment to relax.

Then, ask yourself the question, "How do I see my body right now?" Take as long as you need to contemplate the answer.

Now, open your eyes. Pick the colored felt pens of our choice and draw a picture of your body as you "see" it now. Do not try to make art or a "pretty picture." This is not an art class, and you are not being judged on your artistic ability or talent. Simply portray how you see your body at this time in your life.

Look at your drawing. Then write about the image you see there.

Benefits: In this activity you pinpoint your true feelings about your body. As your feelings change about your body, you can observe your progress by repeating this exercise and comparing your drawings.

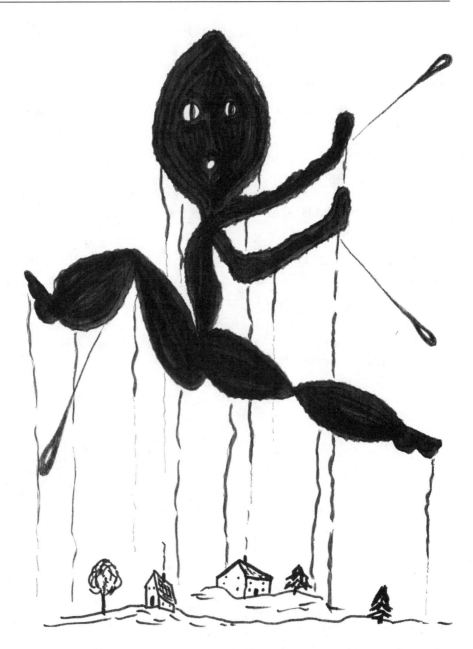

I feel like a balloon-man . . . . full of volatile gas rising out of control. My skin twitches with the fear of being pricked. If pricked I would explode damaging everything around me. I'm rising too fast and swelling beyond my limits. I'm going to explode! My course is bent on destruction.

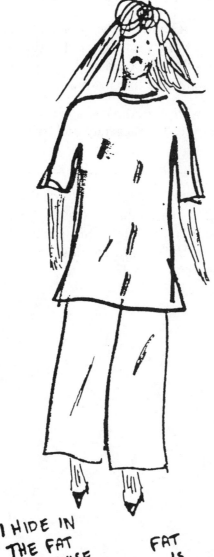

I HIDE IN
THE FAT
BECAUSE   FAT
I AM SAD   IS
                SAD

IF I'M SAD I DON'T CARE
HOW I LOOK   I COVER
        MYSELF UP

LAUGHING AT MYSELF

Draw a page filled with caricatures of your body. Be as silly and outrageous as you like! If you think your legs are fat, then draw them huge like elephant legs. The sillier, the crazier, the better. If you think your body is sagging, then dramatize that in your drawing.

When you are finished, write a short paragraph about how you feel right now. This is the time to really exaggerate and let your humor out.

Benefits: In this exercise we take the heaviness out of body image and weight issues. It helps to have a sense of humor and to be able to laugh about yourself and your negative beliefs. Here, we truly "Lighten Up" and the results are feelings of good will and love for your own self.

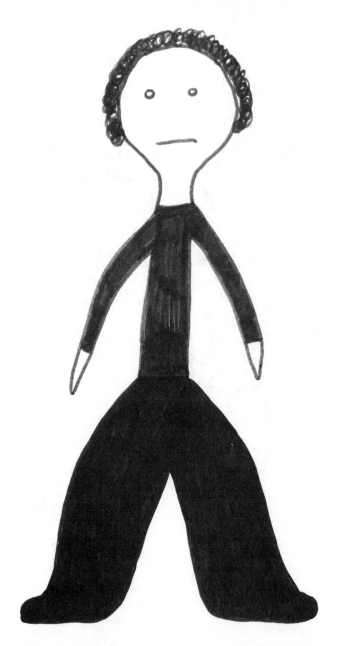

My legs are so dense and heavy I can hardly move. My torso feels like a broomstick growing out of my massive legs and my arms like matchsticks. I can't move fast enough to stay on top of things, and even if I could, my arms are too frail to do anything.

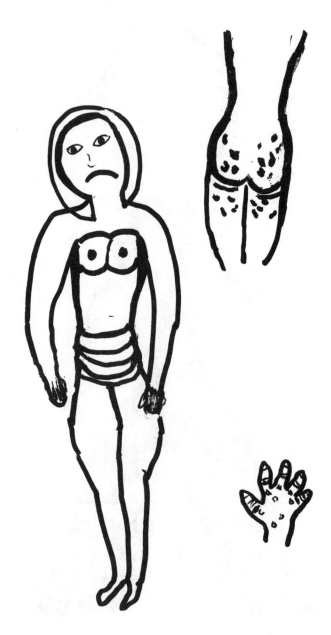

My butt is so bumpy with pockets of fat I look like cottage cheese at the beach. My waist looks like a wrist filled with bangle bracelets. My hands are so spotted and wrinkled and worn they look one hundred years old. My mouth is so bowed it looks like I'm frowning all the time. Poor me!

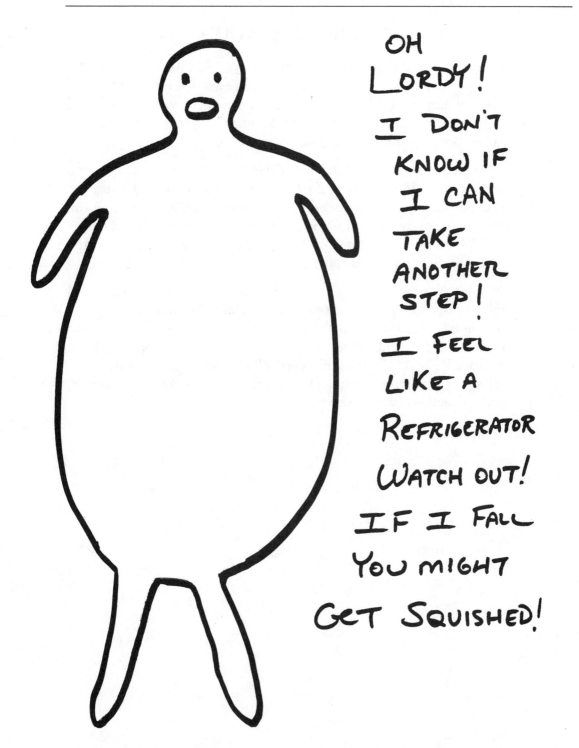

OH LORDY! I DON'T KNOW IF I CAN TAKE ANOTHER STEP! I FEEL LIKE A REFRIGERATOR WATCH OUT! IF I FALL YOU MIGHT GET SQUISHED!

DEEP RELAXATION

In order to bring about any lasting change, you first need to experience your physical body *as it is*. A state of deep relaxation creates the internal environment in which it is possible to reconnect with your physical sensations. By enabling you to "come home" to your body, it allows inner change and healing to take place.

Balanced, rhythmic breathing is probably the oldest and most universal method for entering a state of deep relaxation and for revitalizing the body. By focusing your awareness on your natural breathing rhythm you are able to slow down the internal chatter of the mind and allow the body to fully relax. You are also nourishing yourself through one of your principal life supports—the breath.

In order to do the following exercise, it is important to be in a quiet and private place with no distractions or interruptions. You will be lying down in a simple yoga posture that has been used for thousands of years to relax, revitalize, and balance the flow of energy in the body. It is no coincidence that it is called the "corpse" posture! For in order to deeply relax, it is important to temporarily disconnect from the sights, sounds, and distractions of our everyday world.

NATURAL BREATHING MEDITATION

Lie on your back on a carpeted floor or a firm bed. Elongate your body so that your spine is straight, and you can relax and breathe more fully. Your legs are straight, with your feet about twelve to eighteen inches apart. Your arms are straight and about six to nine inches from your sides. Your palms are facing upwards. Your chin is tipped slightly down toward the chest to elongate the neck and spine. The back of your head is resting comfortably on the floor or bed.

Close your eyes and allow your mind and body to relax. You may want to take a few deep breaths to release any tension. Now, focus your attention on your breathing. Listen to the sound of your inbreath and outbreath.

Observe how you are breathing. Are you breathing through your nose or your mouth? Is the rhythm of your breathing fast or slow? Is your breathing shallow or deep? Notice where you take the breath into your body. Is there more movement in your upper chest or down in your lower abdomen? (You can place your hands on your abdomen or chest to better feel the movement in your body.)

Now, breathe through your nose, inhaling and exhaling in a smooth and effortless rhythm. Slowly let your abdomen, then your rib cage, and finally your upper chest rise and expand, filling up with air. Then, slowly exhale, first from your abdomen, then your rib cage, and lastly your upper chest. Continue listening to the sound of your breath.

As you inhale, feel the oxygen nourishing and refreshing your entire body. As you exhale let the breath carry away tension, worry, and any other "heaviness." Gradually allow your breathing to become deeper, slower, and more rhythmic. Do not force the breathing. Just allow the air to come in and go out in a steady, even flow. As you relax into your body and the natural rhythm of your breathing, let the air breathe you. You may experience feelings of energy, vibrancy, and peacefulness as you breathe deeper and more slowly. Notice how light you feel and how quiet your mind becomes!

JOURNEY THROUGH THE BODY

Next you will take a long, leisurely journey through your body. First read the guidelines carefully and remember them as best you can. Then do the process by lying down comfortably on your back as you practiced in the natural breathing exercise. Do this inner journey through the body very slowly with your eyes closed, paying attention to everything you feel inside.

Imagine that your consciousness is shrinking down to a tiny point of light at the top of your head. You might see it as a tiny flashlight or a lamp to illumine the way. You are now going to travel inside and feel the sensations in each area of your body.

Start at your forehead. Feel the sensations in this area. Do you experience tension or do you feel relaxed? Observe how your forehead feels. Then, slowly move your awareness down your face. Observe the sensations around and behind your eyes, first your left eye, and then your right eye. Do you feel strain or fatigue there? Or is it relaxed? Then move to your nose, cheeks, and sinus area. Observe the sensations there. Are you breathing openly or are you congested? Now slowly move down to your mouth, your chin and jaw. How does this area feel? Is it tense or relaxed? Go inside your mouth and observe the sensations in your tongue, gums, teeth, and other areas there. How does it feel?

Now, travel slowly down to the inside of your throat. How does it feel there? Is your throat open or constricted? Does it feel good or is it sore? Next, check out your neck, both front and back. Is it tense or relaxed? Observe all the sensations there. Now, note the feelings in your shoulders and the joints which connect your arms to your body. Be aware of the right shoulder joint and then the left shoulder joint. How do they feel?

Travel slowly down your arms; first the left arm and then the right. Observe the feeling in your left arm. Start with the upper arm, then move down to the elbow. How do these areas feel? Then notice the sensation in your left forearm and wrist. Be aware of your left hand and check out the palm, the back of the hand, and then each finger. How do they feel? Then repeat the journey, this time traveling down the right arm. Again, start with the upper arm, moving down to the elbow. Notice all the sensations as your awareness moves from one area to the other. Observe the feelings in your right forearm and wrist. Then notice the sensations in your right hand: the palm, the back of the hand, and each finger.

Now, return to your torso. Slowly begin to move your awareness down the front of your body. Observe the feelings in your chest. Does it feel tight and held in? Or does it feel open and expansive? Do your lungs inhale deeply and easily, and exhale as naturally? Do you experience any constriction and difficulty in breathing fully? Be aware of the feelings and sensations in your heart area. Does your heart feel open or constricted?

Next, allow your awareness to travel down the center of your body to your stomach and digestive system. How does it feel there? Does it feel energized and expansive, or does it feel full and sluggish? Now, move down your abdomen to the area of the bladder and intestines. What sensations are you aware of? Is there a sense of movement or "holding on"? If you feel sensations in the abdominal area but are not sure which organ is causing them, simply note the sensations and the location. Next, move down to your genitals. Observe any sensations or feelings you experience there.

Now, return to the back of your neck and observe the sensations in your upper back and shoulders. Is there tension and soreness there? Or do you feel loose and relaxed? Move slowly down your spine and the middle of your back. Then observe feelings in your lower back and pelvic area. Is there any stiffness or soreness? Do you feel comfortable and relaxed? Continue down to the base of your spine, your anus, and buttocks. What kinds of sensations do you experience there?

Finally, move down your legs. Begin with the left pelvic joint and travel down your left leg. Observe the sensations in your left thigh. Then move down to your left knee. Are these areas tense or relaxed? Move gradually down the calf to the ankles checking out all the sensations. Lastly, move down into your left foot: the top, the sole, and then each toe. How does the foot feel? Now, repeating this journey, move your awareness gradually down your right leg. Start with the right pelvic joint and check out the sensations in your right thigh. Then move down to the knee. How does this area feel? Then move down your right calf to the ankle. Then check out your right foot: the top, the sole, and then each toe. What sensations do you feel there?

Allow yourself to relax even more deeply and do a quick review of this inner journey through the body. Make a mental note of any areas of stress, pain, or discomfort.

When you inhale, consciously send the energy of the breath to those areas of your body. Take plenty of time. In this way you are nourishing the parts of your body that need tender loving care.

Benefits: In order to bring about any lasting change in your weight, shape, or body image, it is first essential to get to *know* your body. The Natural Breathing Meditation and the Journey Through the Body are intended to help you become more aware of your body and what is going on inside of you. When used regularly, these meditations help you to listen to your body's messages—sensations and inner feelings. This is the first step in making friends with your body. Once you begin to make friends with your body, you can begin to feel truly at home in your body.

You will be using the Natural Breathing Meditation and Journey Through the Body repeatedly throughout this book. Many have found it extremely helpful to have an audio tape of this narration. For this purpose, you may want to use Lucia's audio cassette, *Well-Being Journal Meditations*. The meditations are accompanied by original music. To order this cassette, contact: INNERWORKS, 1341 Ocean Ave., #100, Santa Monica, CA 90401. If you prefer to record the exercises in your voice for your own personal use, you have our permission.

DRAWING HOW MY BODY FEELS

Do the Natural Breathing Meditation and Body Journey. Ask yourself:

How does my body feel right now?

Close your eyes and experience the feelings inside your body.

Now, with your non-dominant hand, draw a freehand picture of your body which expresses how it feels. Remember, you are making this drawing only for *you*—it is not for public exhibition. The drawing can be very simple (a cartoon, stick figure, or silhouette). You are getting in touch with how your body feels to you and then expressing this through drawing. Use different colored pens to color in areas of the body where you have particularly strong sensations. You may also include any emotions and feelings that arise. Write the names of sensations and feelings in or around the drawing.

Benefits: Here is a tool for further developing your ability to visualize. It is a means for using drawing in the service of awareness and well-being, a way to sensitize you and help you communicate with your body. By labeling physical sensations and emotions, this exercise gets you further in touch with your body and what it is saying to you.

TALKING WITH MY BODY

Look at your Body Drawing from the previous activity, or draw a new one. Look at each area you have labeled or colored.

Now, pretend that your Body Drawing can speak to you. Have a conversation with your body on paper. Write the questions with your dominant hand, and let the body answer with your non-dominant hand. Use a different color pen in each hand. Do not preplan the dialogue. Let it happen spontaneously.

Do not worry about spelling, grammar, or vocabulary in writing with the non-dominant hand. It often speaks and writes in a language of its own, disregarding rules and conventions. Although your non-dominant handwriting may be awkward, slow, and barely legible at first, as you continue the initial frustrations and difficulties will lessen.

When the conversation is over, reread what you and your body had to say to each other. Write down what this reveals to you. If your body has stated problems, complaints, worries, etc., write down what you can do about them.

Benefits: Paying attention to our physical sensations is the first step in improving our body image and reclaiming our natural body. Body conversations can be invaluable tools for establishing a working relationship with your body. They help you shift from the rational left brain into the creative right brain where you can experience breakthroughs in old patterns and access your intuitive wisdom for problem-solving.

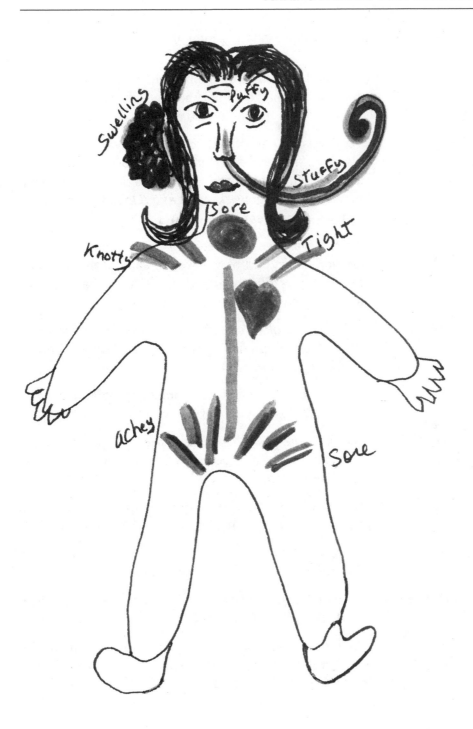

BODY DIALOGUE

ME: High and hi. What's been up or down with you today? I know you've had a lot of changes & you woke up feeling like you were getting a cold.

BODY: *Yes, I was feeling scared and awful—my nose was stuffed up—my throat sore and my whole body felt tight and achy. Another cold again. But instead of feeling sorry for me & letting me get sicker you asked John for a massage. Boy was that great.*

ME: It really was—we saw pictures & felt feelings and talked about the hurt part of us—like the ear and the nose and the sinuses as John massaged and released the sore, tight area and muscles. Ear, what happened?

EAR: *It felt like an old piece of broccoli that finally blew out. It was black & green & yellow. I felt a drop of potion— magic potion and I felt better.*

ME: I know you do—it felt like something dark was being removed. Nose—what happened to you?

NOSE: *I can breathe now—out came a stream of green mucus— breath of fire like a dragon. It's gone now. We can breathe together—happy.*

ME: I'll say! We feel so relaxed, our breathing is so peaceful and unobstructed. What about you, sinus and forehead?

SINUS: *I'm feeling better—I was puffy & full of mucus. Now I feel less full. But my forehead is still tight.*

FOREHEAD: *I want my forehead rubbed. The tightness will go away then. Everything feels stuck up here.*

ME: Well, that's not too bad. By tomorrow we should be much better. We're just in the process of healing. How's the neck, shoulders and back?

NECK/ *SHOULDERS/* *BACK:*	*We're great – feeling great – not sore and tight anymore – soft, relaxed – healing – need to rest so we can move and be a happy body again.*
ME:	Well, I think I learned a lot today. Take care of myself and don't be afraid to ask for help. Pay attention to the messages behind the pictures in my mind. Take special care and nurture myself instead of giving myself a hard time for being sick and trying to heal.

(Four hours later)

ME:	The body massage and written dialogues have gotten me in touch with the pictures and symbols in my mind of past situations that needed forgiveness and compassion. The allergy/cold condition has completely dissolved with the exception of a slight heaviness in the forehead. Thank you body and mind for uniting and healing one another.

HOW I WOULD LIKE TO FEEL

Using your non-dominant hand, draw a picture of how you would like your body to feel. Include colors and shapes to signify vitality and health.

Then with your non-dominant hand, describe how it feels to be in the body you just pictured.

Benefits: Drawing and dialoguing about how you would like to feel will help you get in touch with that state so that it becomes a reality. Remember to work with the idea of the perfect body which nature intended for you *right now* with your lifestyle and stage of development, rather than the body of someone much younger and leading an entirely different life.

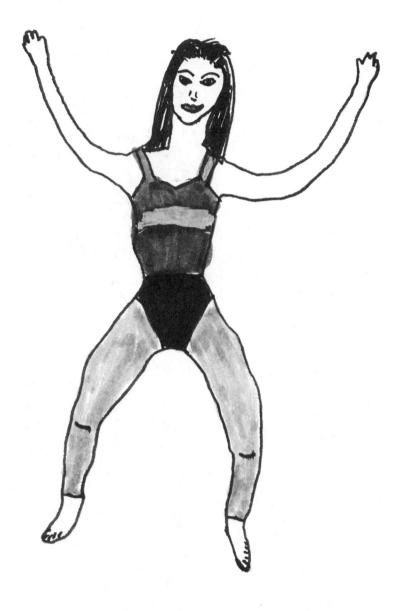

I jump & fly with joy. In a moment I am lifted off my feet. I am in the air. I am in ecstasy. The dancer & dance are one. I move in and through the body. I delight in the form that is my friend and home.

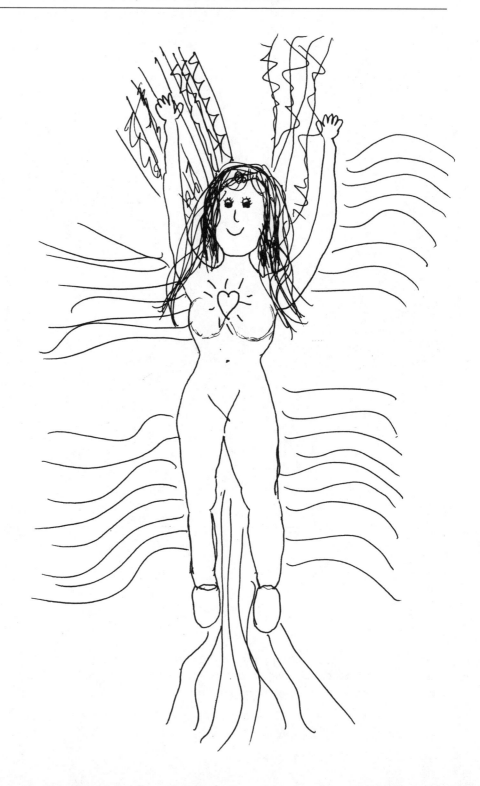

I am powerful.
I am a winner.
I am free & full.

I am whole & in balanced.

I am open & Radiant.

I am loving & I am loved.
Love, growth, spiritual
Light, energy, vibrant
Visable, successful

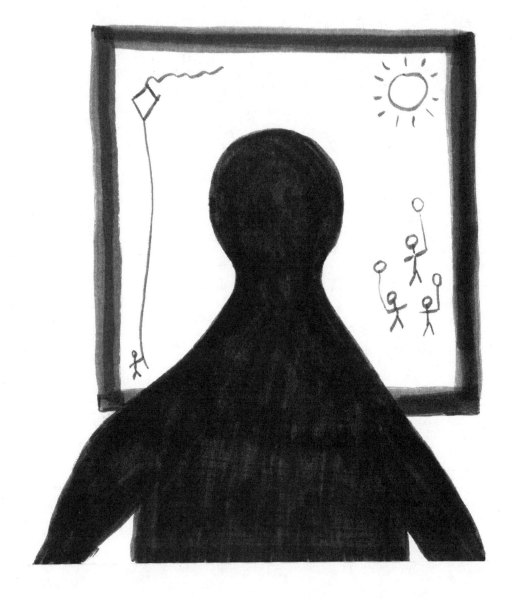

CHAPTER THREE

Eat Something, You'll Feel Better

The greatest discovery of any generation is that human beings can alter their lives by altering the attitudes of their minds.

—Albert Schweitzer

"Eat something, you'll feel better." Is this a familiar refrain? Did you grow up in a household where food was used as a way to deal with feelings, where difficult emotions were stuffed down with food? If so, you were programmed to use food as a narcotic. You were taught that food was a magic potion that would numb your physical and emotional pain. The relief is only temporary, however, and the feelings resurface only to be forced down again and again with food. This cycle can lead to weight and health problems, in addition to low self-esteem, guilt, and shame.

One way you can change this programming—that food will remove pain—is by learning to accept and honor all of your feelings. Your feelings are an important part of who you really are. Feelings are never right or wrong, good or bad; they simply exist. When feelings are accepted and expressed safely, they can be great allies. As you found in Chapter 2, listening to feelings that live in the body helps us contact our instinctual wisdom. For it is in our "gut instincts" that we carry a deep inner knowing which can help guide our lives. Our feelings can act as our personal radar for detecting which people and situations are nurturing for us, and which ones are unhealthy. When our feelings are blocked, however, we lose touch with our instinctual wisdom. This leaves us feeling empty and unfulfilled inside. When we stop listening to our own inner truth, we can easily become addicted to substances, activities, or dogmas. We can also

43

become dependent upon others in our search for an outer force to guide our lives.

A major premise in psychological treatment for weight control is that emotions which are repeatedly suppressed or repressed with food literally get "stuffed" in the body. Food becomes the "cork" which keeps the emotions bottled up. Obsessive/compulsive eating patterns such as overeating, binging and purging (bulimia), and deprivation (anorexia), are all signs of "emotional starvation," and a hungry heart that is longing to be fed. Food here is used as a sorry substitute for love and self-acceptance.

Self-acceptance begins with accepting our feelings. We all have them and that is a part of being human. However, when we deny our feelings, those feelings "have us." The more we judge them, fight them, or cover them up, the more they gain control beneath the surface. Feelings are forms of energy, and that energy does not go away by simply ignoring it. Instead, our imprisoned emotional energy can either burst out of control in unconscious behavior (acting out), or remain locked in the body where it can lead to physical and emotional distress or illness.

In the following exercises you will be guided toward a loving acceptance of the full spectrum of your feelings. As you express your true self safely and creatively through drawing and writing, the need to tranquilize your feelings with food diminishes. As you release buried emotional energy through creative expression, you are likely to experience more physical energy, a heightened level of vitality, and a new experience of your body.

If sensitive issues such as childhood abuse come to the surface while doing this work, we urge you to seek professional help. These issues are not within the scope of this book and should not be dealt with alone or in isolation. A strong support system is essential for helping you with your healing.

DRAWING YOUR FEELINGS OUT

Allow yourself to sit quietly for a moment and focus your awareness on your natural breathing rhythm. As you relax, begin tuning into your feelings. Allow yourself to experience them fully. If your feelings had color and shape, what would it be? If your feelings could make sounds, what sounds would they be? What kind of rhythm would they have? Do your feelings have a texture or a pattern? Are your feelings hot, warm, or cold?

Now, using your non-dominant hand, draw your feelings out on paper. Choose the colors that feel right for you. Allow yourself to draw spontaneously without judgment or concern for the final outcome. Have fun exploring and experimenting, and let your drawing be a process. Your picture does not have to look like anything in the outer world. It is fine to scribble, doodle, and make abstract shapes, lines, and patterns. Allow your drawing to be an outward expression of your inner world.

Benefits: In this exercise you learn to express your inner feelings through the language of art. It also allows you to access the creative and intuitive powers of your right brain by drawing with your non-dominant hand.

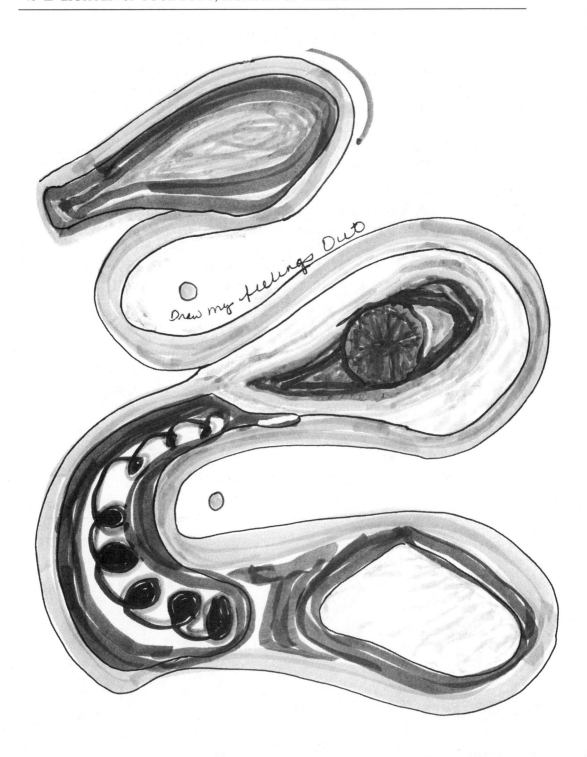

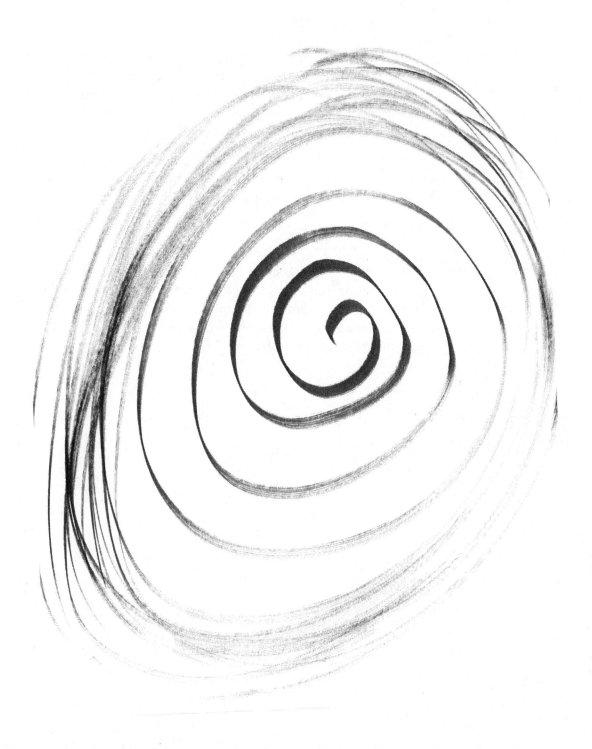

I'M FEELING SO HUNGRY.....

Think about a time when you were feeling really hungry, and for some reason you were prevented from eating. You may have had to wait a long time to be served at a restaurant, you may have been in a job siutation which kept you working beyond mealtime, or you may have been traveling and unable to find a grocery store or diner.

How did you feel? What did you say? What did you do? Draw a picture of yourself feeling hungry. You may include captions or word balloons which tell how you felt and/or what you said.

When you think about being hungry, what feelings come up?

Benefits: This exercise is designed to demonstrate the connection between eating and emotions. Hunger may bring up infantile emotions as it triggers our primitive instinct for survival and nourishment. Just ask anyone who has ever served hungry customers in a busy restaurant!

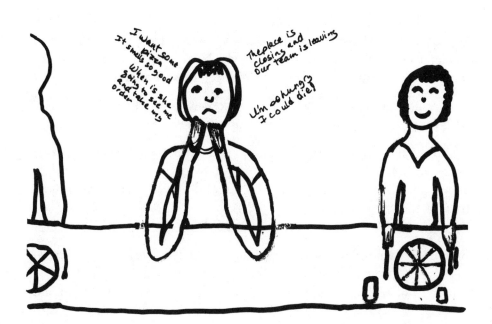

I'M SO MAD I COULD.....

Take a moment to sit quietly and relax. Allow yourself to breathe naturally. Contemplate what the word "anger" means to you. When do you feel angry? In what situations, around which people? Are there particular foods and beverages you associate with feelings of anger?

Now, using any colors, shapes, forms, or designs, draw a picture of "anger" with your non-dominant hand. Let yourself and your colored markers go!

When the drawing is complete, have a conversation with "anger" using both hands. Let "anger" write with your non-dominant hand. What does anger have to say to you? Why does it feel that way? What can you do to help each other?

Benefits: Many of us have been taught that it is wrong to be angry. One way that we often try to relieve our anger is to eat, instead of feeling or expressing the emotion. The next time you are angry, try pounding a pillow instead of stuffing your body with food.

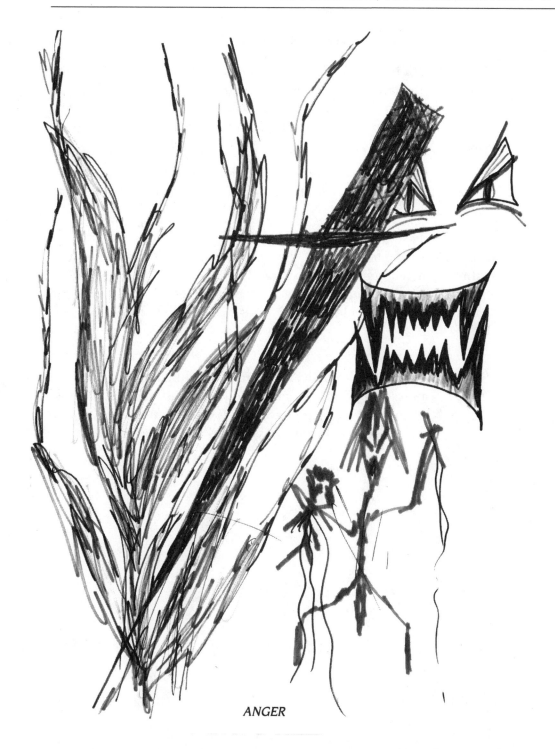

ANGER

I'M SO SAD AND LONELY

Allow yourself to sit quietly and relax. Begin to breathe naturally. Now, remember the last time you felt sad. Tune into the feeling of sadness. Are there certain people or situations that tend to make you sad? Are there particular foods and beverages you associate with feelings of sadness?

Using your non-dominant hand, draw a picture of a person who is very sad and lonely. Draw them as unhappy, as teary, and as woeful as possible.

When you have finished the drawing, have a written conversation with this person using both hands. Allow the sad and lonely person to write with your non-dominant hand. What do they have to tell you? Why is he or she so sad and lonely? What foods or beverages do they like to eat or drink when they feel that way? What can you do to help them feel better?

Benefits: There are alternatives to eating and drinking our emotions away. As we explore sadness and loneliness and their causes, we may see the options available to freeing ourselves from any self-destructive behavior associated with these emotions.

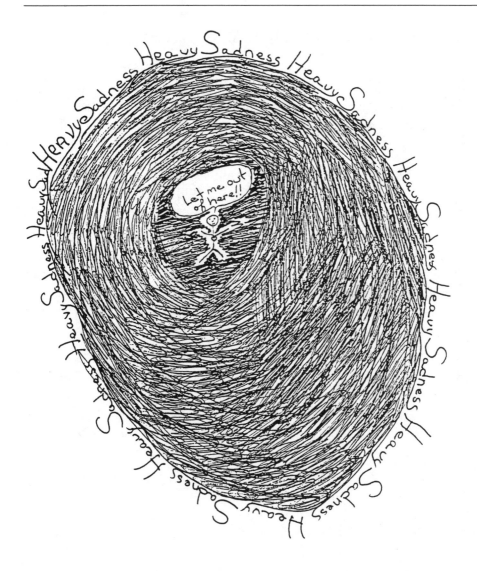

Ohhhhhhh . . . . . I'm soooooooo saaaaaaaaad. I want to crawl into bed with a bowl of ice cream and a pan of hot fudge. I will eat and sleep this sadness away. I am so sad I don't even know the reason. Now, that's sad.

But it's too early to go to bed. And I don't have any ice cream. Maybe I'll walk to Haagen Daaz . . . or maybe I'll walk to the park . . . I don't want to be with any of my friends . . . so maybe I'll walk to the park and look at some strangers.

I'M SO SICK AND TIRED

Sit quietly, relax, and begin to breathe naturally. Contemplate the last time you felt exhausted and in the throes of despair—completely "sick and tired" of things. Are there situations or people in your life which provoke this feeling? Are there particular foods and beverages which you associate with feelings of exhaustion and despair?

Using your non-dominant hand, draw a picture of a person who is feeling very "sick and tired." You can make it simple or as dramatic as you like.

When you have finished the drawing, have a written conversation with this "sick and tired" person using both hands. Allow the "sick and tired" person to write with your non-dominant hand. What does he or she have to tell you? Why are they so exhausted and depressed? What foods or beverages does the "sick and tired" person like to eat or drink? What can you do to help them feel better?

Benefits: In this exercise, we explore feelings of exhaustion and depression in order to better understand their causes. This, in turn, may open us up to more constructive ways of dealing with these feelings rather than taking them out on our bodies by overeating.

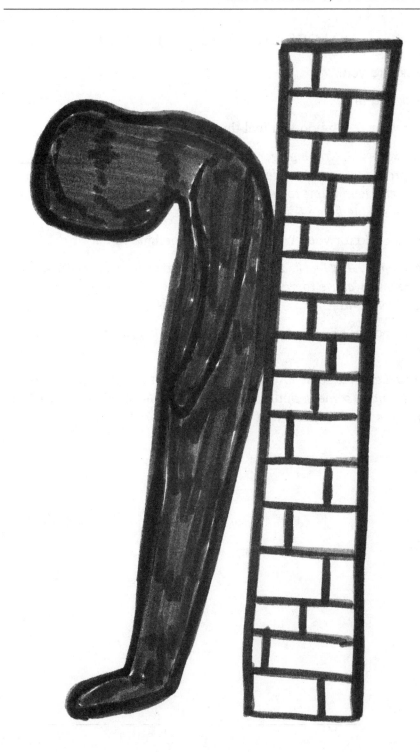

DIALOGUE WITH SICK AND TIRED

Hi! Who are you?

I'm sick and tired . . . .

What's wrong? Why do you feel this way?

I don't know . . . Nothing seems to work anymore. Life is the pits. So many problems and obstacles. I don't like my job, my car doesn't run and my girlfriend wants to leave. I don't want to go on. There's no point to life. It's a big game & I'm sick of playing.

What can I do for you? Would you like something to eat or drink?

I'm not hungry, but I'd like a big bowl of potato chips. I'd also like a beer. Not too much 'cause there's not too much room left. Need some room for ice cream later.

Is there another way that I could make you feel better without giving you food?

You could give me some love & understanding. It gets so hopeless sometimes & I need some support, something to believe in. I could believe in love. It's the only thing that makes sense to me.

I'M SO SCARED I COULD . . .

Sit quietly, focus on your natural breathing and allow yourself to relax. As you relax, contemplate the feeling of fear. What does the word "fear" mean to you? When do you feel fearful? Around which people? In what situations? Are there particular foods or beverages you associate with feelings of fear?

Now, using your non-dominant hand, draw a picture of "fear." Use any colors, shapes, and designs that you wish. When you are finished, contemplate the picture.

Then have a conversation with the picture using both hands. Let "fear" write with your non-dominant hand. What does fear have to say? What do you have to say to fear? Conclude the conversation by agreeing on ways you and fear can work together.

Benefits: Our fears are often based on lack of proper information or the loss of others' approval. Here, you can safely explore your fears. You can reclaim the fearful part of yourself, and turn it into a friend who works with you, not against you.

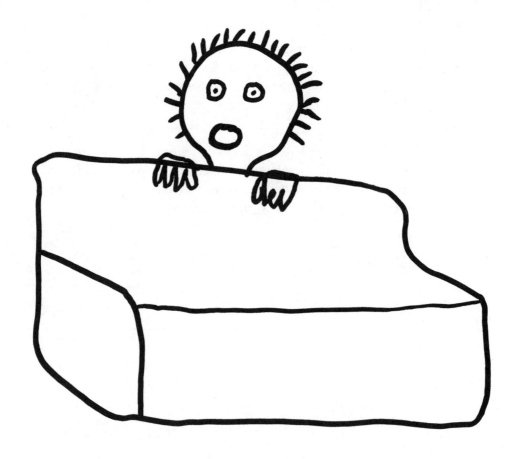

FEAR

DIALOGUE WITH FEAR

Who are you?

Fear.

How do you feel?

SCARED!!

What's going on?

They're gonna get me.

Who?

Monsters.

Why?

I dunno. They like to eat children.

Did you see the monsters?

No, they're around the corner. I can hear them.

What can I do to help you?

Chase the monsters away.

Why do you think they will be scared of me?

You're big.

Aren't they big too?

Yah. I guess so.

You have never seen them?

Well, no, I don't think so.

Why don't you get up and go see if the monsters are really there?

Well, I don't know.

Remember, I'm big. You don't have anything to be scared of.

I don't know.

Come on, I'll hold your hand and we'll go see together. Monsters are scared of little boys.

Really?

Yes.

LET'S GO!

I'M SO HAPPY I COULD . . . . . .

Sit quietly, relax, and focus on your natural breathing. Now, contemplate the feeling of happiness. When was the last time you felt really happy? Are there certain situations which make you happy? Do you feel happy around certain people? Are there certain foods and beverages you associate with feelings of happiness?

Using your non-dominant hand, draw a picture of joy or happiness.

When you have finished the drawing, have a written conversation with happiness using both hands. Allow happiness to write with your non-dominant hand. What does happiness have to tell you? How can it become more a part of your life?

Benefits: For many of us happiness has been equated with certain foods. Eating was a "quick fix" to feel better when difficult situations or emotions arose. Knowing what *really* makes you happy is the first step toward creating a nurturing lifestyle. The goal is to experience contentment and satisfaction. This is done by filling your life with whatever makes you truly happy, rather than filling your body up with food as a substitute for happiness.

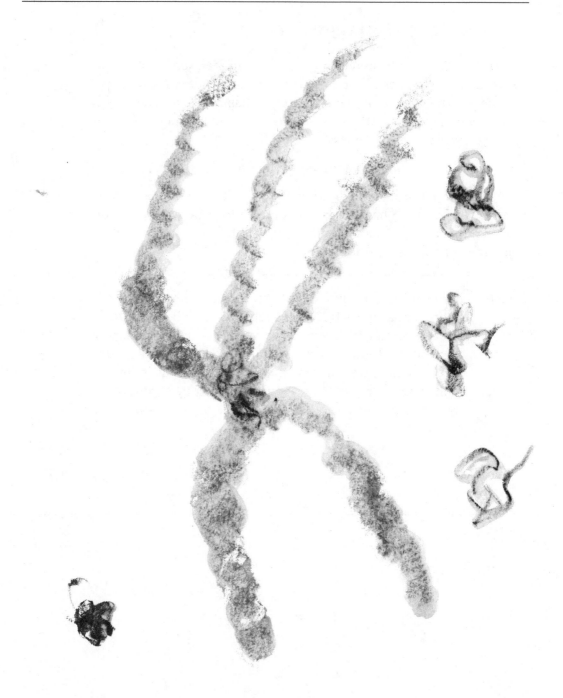

JOY

DIALOGUE WITH JOY

Who are you?

I am JOY.

How do you feel?

Great! I feel like I'm going to jump right out of my skin! I can hardly contain myself.

Why do you feel this way?

Because everything is going my way. The way of JOY! I am always here ready to burst forth but you worry so much about appearances. You keep me locked in a room because you don't know what to do with me!

What can I do to feel you more often?

Don't be afraid of me. I'm your best friend. I make you feel really good. It's so simple. Everything is in your life at every moment. You just have to see it!

LOVE

Sit quietly and focus on your natural breathing. Relax and contemplate the feeling of love. When was the last time you felt love? Are there certain situations or people in your life around which it is easier to feel love? What foods and beverages do you associate with feelings of love?

Using your non-dominant hand, draw a picture of "love." You can make it simple or as dramatic as you like. Use as many colors as you wish.

When you have finished the drawing, have a written conversation with "love" using both hands. Allow love to write with your non-dominant hand. What does love have to tell you? Why is it feeling that way? What does love have to teach you?

Benefits: In this exercise, we explore feelings of love. Love is not only the best nourishment for the body and soul, but it has the power to heal any difficult emotions we find ourselves struggling with.

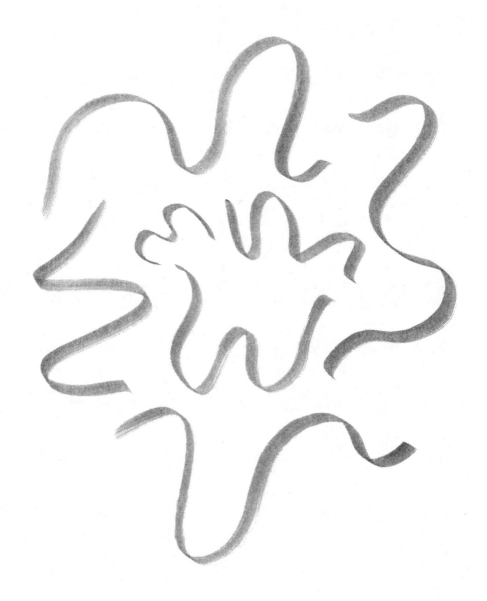

LOVE

DIALOGUE WITH LOVE

Who are you?

I am Love.

What does it feel like to be Love?

Radiant, courageous, and full of light.

How can I feel more of you in my life?

Life is a gift. Be content with what you have been given and don't be attached to things which cannot bring you happiness. Be grateful for each day as it comes & live one day at a time.

Be happy! Your life will be full of love if you learn how to serve. Above all else, recognize that you are worthy of love, from others and from yourself. This is the greatest truth & the solution to all your problems. It's right under your nose! Go for it! I love you!

HOW I FEEL ABOUT FOOD

In your journal, write down the word "FOOD." Without stopping to think, immediately write down all the words you associate with "FOOD." Write quickly, off the top of your head. Do not ponder over it too much. Let the words flow freely, each word triggering the next in a chain reaction. Write as long as you wish.

When you have finished, look over what you have written. With your non-dominant hand, write down any observations or feelings you had while making the list of words you associate with "FOOD."

Benefits: Our attitudes and habits about food are shaped in early childhood by our parents and others in our lives. If you have unhealthy eating or drinking patterns, it is important to get to the root of these attitudes in order to change them. This exercise can help you explore your unconscious attitudes about food and nourishment. It is especially helpful to deal with these attitudes if eating or drinking has become a problem area for you, such as in the case of overeating, alcoholism, and bulimia.

<u>Food</u> Steak   Party

Yipeeeee!!! fat good   nourishment

icecream beer heavy thighs

 hotdog

Alone Silence brunch

 Starving

 Mexican no money

Sidewalk
cafés   Stomach

 Onions Biafra

Swedish McDonalds
meatballs Cooking

eat your vegetables

 cigarettes

fish/ocean/swim/sun

FOODS AND MOODS

Make a list of your favorite foods and beverages. Now, using your non-dominant hand, write a word which describes how you feel inside when you think of each particular food or drink. Review your list of foods/drinks and feelings. Write down any observations you have.

What is the significance of food in your life? Is eating related to any particular emotions? What about drinking? Do you crave particular foods or beverages when you are in certain moods? If so, what are they? If possible, observe this pattern when it happens and try to write about it at the time (or as soon as possible).

Benefits: Here is an opportunity to become more aware of your attitudes, feelings, and habits regarding physical nourishment. It can help you understand the deeper emotional significance that food has in your life beyond physical sustenance.

Note: These exercises have been very helpful for individuals with substance abuse problems. If you suffer with substance abuse of any kind (drugs, cigarettes, alcohol, etc.) modify the exercise and focus on the substance in question rather than food.

FOODS AND MOODS

Pasta	Weighted-down
Steamed vegetables	Content
Salad	Peaceful
Tomatoes	Fiery
Black Bean soup	Energized
Potato chips	Anxious
Lasagna	Satisfied
Brown rice	Healthy
Pizza	Angry
Black Tea	Unruffled
Carrot juice	Light
Lentil soup	Nurtured
Cheese	Clogged
Cookies	Happy
Ice cream	Depressed
Orange juice	Nourished
Mangos	Adventurous
Coffee	Stimulated

WATCHING MY EATING PATTERNS

Observe your eating patterns for one week. Do you tend to eat quickly, or in a leisurely manner? Do you generally enjoy the experience of eating? Do you eat what you want to eat, or what you think you ought to eat? Do you ask your body what it needs, or are your food choices prompted by emotions? Do you make enough time for eating as a separate activity, or do you set up your schedule so that there is never time to digest and enjoy a meal? Do you often feel anxious or distracted while eating?

Where do you usually eat your meals? Restaurants, at home or in the office? Do you eat alone or with others? Do you generally feel satisfied after a meal, or do you find yourself craving more food after you are finished? Each day write down highlights or insights about your eating patterns.

At week's end, look over your observational notes. Write about any reactions you have and any recurring patterns you see.

How would you like to experience eating in the future? What would be nourishing to your body and soul? What would you do to make eating a pleasurable and satisfying part of your day? What would make eating a delight for your senses and emotions? Using your imagination picture in your mind how you want to experience eating. Feel that experience in your body. Then act as if your vision were a reality. Write about it in the first person, present tense.

Benefits: In this exercise you are encouraged to become more conscious of your eating habits. As you observe yourself and become more aware of what you are doing, you then have the freedom to choose a more nourishing and satisfying way of eating. Food can become a wonderful gift for which you are deeply grateful, and eating a special time which you honor and respect.

MY EATING PATTERNS

All last week I ate too fast. I hardly gave myself a chance to swallow one mouth full before shoveling in another. Needless to say, I didn't take the time to chew properly.

I was often distracted when I ate—thinking about work or the next project, reading the paper, watching TV, or talking. I didn't focus on the act of eating itself, and honor and be thankful for the nourishment I was taking into my body. Eating was an unconscious and repetitive act. I did not really taste, savor, or appreciate the *food* I put into my mouth. I began to wonder why I should spend so much time preparing healthy, tasty food if I don't eat it properly.

HOW I'D LIKE TO EAT

I eat my food with great awareness and appreciation. My dining time is a sacred time to me, just like sleeping and meditation. When I eat I just eat. I do not read or think about the concerns of the day. I eat slowly and chew my food thoroughly so I can enjoy it more and aid my digestion. I tend to eat less when I eat slowly, not stuffing my mouth to ease my anxiety. Food is sacred and I treat it as such. By food my body is sustained and all of my cells are nourished. Through food I receive all the energy I need to perform my daily tasks. Because of food, I am alive.

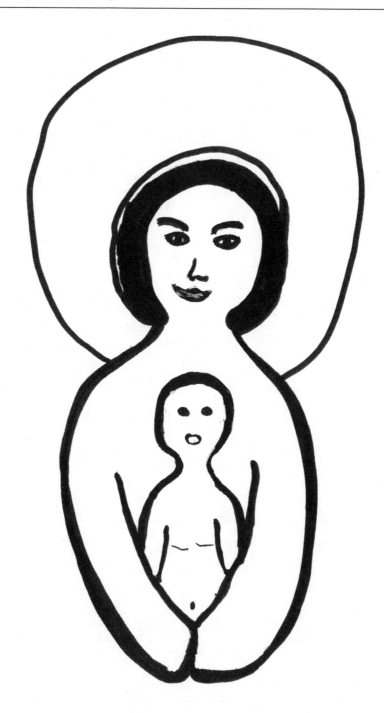

CHAPTER FOUR

Finding the Nurturing Parent
Feeding the Child Within

*It's what we all wanted when we were children—to be loved
and accepted exactly as we were then, not when we got
taller or thinner or prettier . . . and we still want it . . . but
we aren't going to get it from other people until we can get
it from ourselves.*

—Louise Hay

The image of a nurturing parent tenderly feeding a little child brings
warmth to our hearts. It is an ancient archetype symbolizing unconditional love. The theme is timeless and appears in the art of all cultures.
Museums throughout the world are filled with paintings of the Madonna
and child or mothers with their infants.

Although artistic renditions of unconditional love abound, the "real
thing" is rare in our world. We all need love and acceptance in order to
thrive. Love is our natural birthright. Few of us, however, grew up in
families where we were accepted for ourselves, exactly as we were. Instead, most of us were raised on a diet of criticism and conditional "love."
This diet creates the "hole in the soul" referred to so frequently in
twelve-step recovery literature. Addictive behavior is a misguided attempt
to fill this emptiness by numbing the pain of the Inner Child who feels
unloved. As we continue to seek the parental love we so deeply needed
and did not receive in childhood and adolescence, we often turn to food.
However, when food is used as a substitute for love or for the Nurturing Parent, it does not truly nurture, and in fact, may lead to weight and
health problems.

Overeating and extra weight may also serve the unconscious need for
protection. For many of us "inadequate" parenting included emotional
and physical abuse. We did not have protective parents who respected

and guarded our vulnerability as children. The very people who were in the role of caretakers betrayed our trust. Without a good example of protective parenting, we never learned to protect ourselves from invasion or violence. In such cases, extra weight serves as insulation and protection from the outside world, including protection from sexual advances. Weight can distance us from intimate relationships in which getting too close is equated with getting hurt.

The paradox of all of this is that out of loneliness we go in search of the "perfect" relationship—someone who will love us the way we wished our parents had loved us. The results are often disappointing as the real issue has not been addressed. The wounds of childhood have not been healed.

There is only one cure: self-love. As long as we continue looking for love in all the wrong places—outside—we will experience emptiness and despair. As long as we search outside ourselves, wandering around like orphaned children looking for someone to love us, we will remain lost and discontent. Everyone will appear as a good parent or a bad parent, and sometimes the same person will be both. As we wait for love to come to us from others, our hearts may wither from lack of use. Instead, we need to start loving ourselves right now. For until we truly love ourselves, we will not be able to truly love others or receive their love in return.

There is an unlimited supply of love available to us from our own Inner Self. Once we experience this Higher Power within, we can then take up the task of reparenting ourselves and healing the pains of childhood that have left us wounded, homeless—severed from our own bodies and souls.

This task of reparenting ourselves is especially challenging for those of us who suffered childhood abuse, be it emotional, physical, or sexual. According to some experts in the field, 90% of us received inadequate parenting. In fact, the notion of a happy childhood is clearly a myth for many of us in this day and age.

In private counseling and in workshops, clients often ask, "With a horrible childhood like mine, how will I ever find a loving relationship? I don't even know what one looks like." There is only one answer to this question: Create a loving relationship with yourself. Become, for yourself, the loving and protective parents you never had. The response is generally, "This is the hardest thing I've ever had to do." It is not easy, but it is possible. And more than that, it is necessary if we are ever to know real inner peace.

So how do we learn to love our own selves? How do we reparent ourselves? First, we can take healing into our own hands by giving it over to our own Higher Power which we call the Inner Self. This term reinforces the fact that the power of love is within us. It is not an external being who is "superior" to us and one who might punish us for not doing the right thing. The Inner Self is our own inexhaustible source of love, wisdom, guidance, and courage.

Next, we can begin to get in touch with the "family" of characters who live inside of us today: the Critical, Nurturing, and Protective Parents, as well as the Inner Child who is hungry for love and attention. In this chapter you will learn to recognize and deal with the overbearing self-critical voice within, and cultivate a loving Inner Parent who can nurture you and protect you from harm.

> *Within you there is a stillness and a sanctuary to*
> *which you can retreat at any time and be yourself.*
>
> —Herman Hesse

"BE GOOD AND I'LL GIVE YOU A COOKIE"

As a child did you often hear, "Eat all of your dinner then you can have dessert"? What foods were presented to you as your reward for being good? Cookies? Ice cream? Candy? Special food treats? Make a list of these rewards in one column.

When you are finished with the list, look at the rewards. Why were you being rewarded? Were you rewarded for being yourself or for being "good"? Now, next to the rewards list, make a second list of the behavior for which you were given each reward.

Now, with your non-dominant hand, draw a picture of yourself receiving one of the rewards in your list. Let the picture speak about how it feels in captions and word balloons around the figure.

Benefits: As children we are often rewarded for doing something "good" rather than being loved for who we are. This often creates lifelong patterns of behavior aimed at pleasing others in order to receive love. This exercise lets us examine the childhood roots of our associations with food, rewards, and pleasing behavior.

REWARDS	BEHAVIOR
Candy	Stop crying
Cookies	Help with the dishes
Seconds on dinner	Don't talk at the table
My favorite dinner	Clean your room
Apple Pie	Make your bed
Dessert	Eat all your spinach
Popcorn	Sit still (at the movies)
Ice cream	Do your homework
Go out for pizza	Get good grades
Kool aid	Mow the lawn
Popsicle	Help dad with the gardening
Soda	Rake the leaves

GO TO YOUR ROOM WITHOUT DINNER!

As a child were you deprived of food as a form of punishment? Maybe you were sent to your room without supper, or were not given dessert for not finishing your food. Think of all of the various ways in which you were punished for "bad" behavior by being deprived of food.

Using your non-dominant hand draw a picture of yourself in a situation in which you were deprived of food as a child.

Now, allow your picture to speak. Have a dialogue with the child in the picture. Allow the child to write with your non-dominant hand. Ask the child what it did to receive this punishment. What food has it been deprived of? How does it feel?

Benefits: Depriving a child of certain foods is a way of controlling behavior. This association can lead to problems in relationships with food and can trigger a variety of eating disorders.

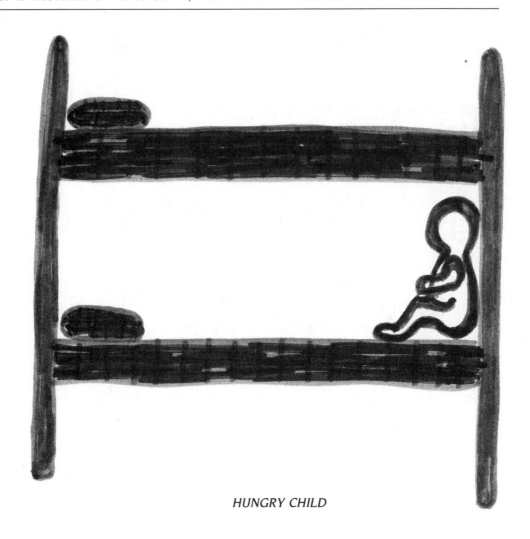

HUNGRY CHILD

DIALOGUE WITH HUNGRY CHILD

Hi! Who are you?

HUNGRY!

What are you doing?

Pouting.

Why?

Mom sent me to my room without dinner.

Why did she do that?

I wouldn't keep quiet at the table.

Is that bad?

No. I just felt good. I couldn't stop talking.

How do you feel?

I'm so mad I could bust! I didn't do anything. I was real happy. Now I'm mad. She is so mean. I hate her when she does that to me.

Why don't we lock the door and play cards? She will never know.

Yeah! I'd like that. Let's do it! But let's keep quiet so she won't know we're having fun!

COOKIE MONSTER

Sit quietly for a moment and close your eyes. Breathe naturally and allow yourself to relax, melting right into the chair.

Pretend that there is a little, round "goodie goblin" hiding somewhere in your body. This "goodie goblin" lives only to eat. It is a food addict. Imagine the goblin stuffing its mouth with lots and lots of food. Imagine it getting bigger and bigger. What does it look like? Is it male or female? What is it wearing? Is it a happy "goodie goblin" or is it sad? Is it frightened or is it angry?

When you have pictured this character clearly in your mind, open your eyes and draw a picture of your "goodie goblin" with your non-dominant hand.

When you have completed your picture, take two different colored felt pens, one for each hand, and have a talk on paper with the "goodie goblin." Using your dominant hand ask the following questions. Let your "goodie goblin" answer with your non-dominant hand.

1) Who are you?
2) How do you feel?
3) What makes you feel that way?
4) What can I do to help you?

Benefits: The impulse to eat may sometimes seem out of control, like a gigantic monster with many heads. However, the willingness to communicate with this part of ourselves can help heal the emptiness we try to fill with food. When given a chance, our inner addicts can turn out to be our best teachers, leading us to better health and a more balanced life.

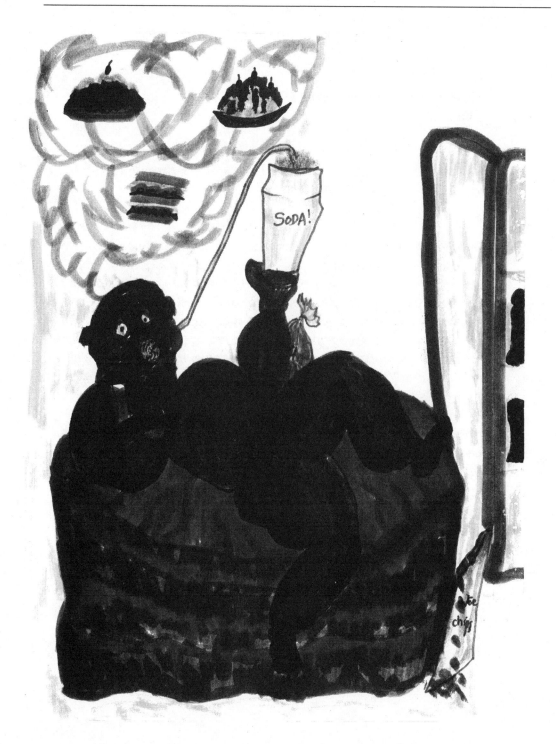

DIALOGUE WITH COOKIE MONSTER

Who are you?

Ah, Ha! I'm the Goodie Goblin! I live only to eat . . . . . to devour . . . . . to consume.

How do you feel?

Insatiable! Needing. Desirous! I feel anguishly empty and I need to be full.

What makes you feel this way?

Deprivation. I'm constantly deprived of those things I need to be full, complete . . . . . love, forgiveness, understanding, God! Sometimes my very existence is stolen from me. I exist! I need to be acknowledged. I'm here. But you! You deny me, or try to. And when my hunger becomes so great even you can't ignore it, you try to appease me by tossing me the bones of acknowledgement. Damn it! Just the bones! You try to stuff my mouth with substitutes. Anything, just to get me to shut up. Well, I'll never shut up! Nothing will suffice but your acceptance that I exist.

What can I do to help you?

Aren't you listening?!?! Of course, you aren't. That's it!! Just listen to me. Listening is the first damn step to acceptance. LISTEN, DON'T STUFF MY MOUTH!!!

CRITICAL PARENT TALKS

Close your eyes and relax. Think of something you do not like about your body or your life, and listen to the critical self-talk that begins to chatter away in your head. These are all the put-downs, judgments, and criticisms you direct toward yourself.

You may hear the critical voice as your own: "I'll never get a date with this face and this body!" Other times it sounds like another person who is whispering in your ear: "You're so fat and ugly! Look at that "spare tire" around your waist. Yukkk! You're hopeless."

Writing with your dominant hand, let your Critical Parent speak. Speak in the third person and let it say whatever it wants about what is wrong with you.

Now, draw a picture of this Critical Parent with your non-dominant hand. Have a written dialogue with the Critical Parent. Let the Critical Parent write with your dominant hand. Answer back with your non-dominant hand. If feelings of anger and outrage come up in the face of your Critical Parent's dialogue, really let yourself express it. It is permissible to use four-letter words, scribble, and write graffiti-like messages.

Benefits: When we were growing up, we often received criticism from our parents or guardians, teachers, coaches, and other authority figures. As we grow up we internalize this criticism and not only project it onto others, but turn it back onto ourselves as well. This exercise gives you an opportunity to observe your critical parent in action and then to answer back, and stand up to it. This dialogue can help you understand how to better nurture yourself and resolve the conflicts arising from your own critical voice.

MY INNER CRITICAL VOICE

You are hopeless.
You never did good in school.
You can't ever find a job you like.
You can't find the right man.
You just haven't got what it takes to succeed.
You eat too much.
You don't ever exercise.
Your body is really out of shape.
You never clean your room.
You are always late for appointments.
You never pay your bills on time.
You procrastinate forever!

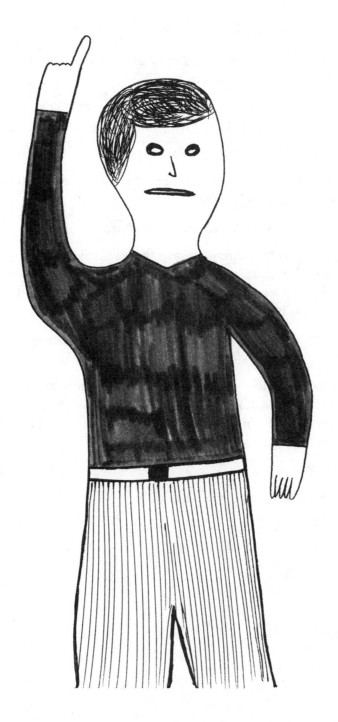

CRITICAL PARENT

DIALOGUE WITH CRITICAL PARENT

CP: *You idiot! Can't you do anything right? You let things slide by and just can't stay on top of your life.*

Me: Wait a minute! Relax! I'm tired of your constant complaining and negativity. Nothing is ever good enough for you.

CP: *That's because you never do anything right.*

Me: With you breathing down my neck it's hard to do anything. Lighten up, for God's sake!

CP: *There you go complaining like a child again.*

Me: No, you listen to me now. I have things I want to do in my life. But I need to be able to learn without being constantly hassled. In my heart I want to have a beautiful, meaningful, and fulfilling life, but you must be willing to work with me.

CP *Well, I try to help you by telling you when you are doing things wrong.*

Me: That's not real help. It's always like, "I told you so." It is not for my best interest. It is for yours. You are afraid of being wrong. Who cares? We will never get anywhere unless we are willing to take chances. Are you up for it?

CP: *I guess so.*

Me: Okay, let's work together on this.

INNER CHILD TALKS

Sit for a moment and think about your Inner Child, or the part of you that is emotional, spontaneous, playful, and creative. It can also be very vulnerable and sensitive. It has a full range of feelings: sadness, fear, hurt, anger, excitement, loneliness, and awkwardness.

Now, draw a picture of your Inner Child with your non-dominant hand.

Then, invite the child to write or print how it feels right now. Use your non-dominant hand.

Benefits: As we grow up our Inner Child is often stifled and pushed underground. However, we can never get rid of our Inner Child—our feelings, our vulnerability, and our creativity. Trying to do away with the Inner Child, instead of expressing it in safe and appropriate ways, can manifest in physical or emotional illness. It can also lead to substance or process addiction in which we try to muffle the cries of the "child in the closet."

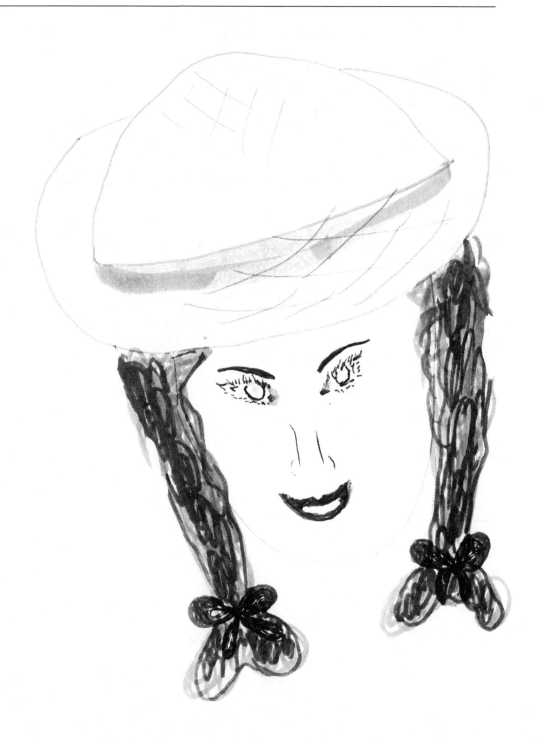

My name is fancy Nancy. I like to play and I like to look chic – I like to mix colors – pink – purples – blues – greens – peach – all the pastels. I like to put pretty colors with pretty fabrics & make pretty clothes. I like to be an artist and paint what I see – flowers – skies, rainbows. I like lace – hats – picnic lunches – I like to sing and dance too. I like myself like this.

FINDING YOUR NURTURING PARENT

Sit quietly for a few moments. Close your eyes and focus on your natural breathing.

Now, imagine that there is a very special character within you called the Inner Nurturer. This character can come in many different forms; i.e., a loving grandparent, a spiritual teacher, a wise guide, a kind nurse, an understanding counselor, a loving friend.

Picture this Inner Nurturer in detail and feel its love and compassion. In your body and your heart, receive the warmth and tender care being given to you.

When you are ready, slowly open your eyes. With your non-dominant hand draw a picture of this Inner Nurturer using whatever colors and shapes come to mind.

Using both hands and two different colored pens, write out a conversation in which you ask for guidance and understanding. Allow this Inner Nurturer to speak to you through your non-dominant hand.

Benefits: In quiet moments we can feel the warmth, protection, and sweetness of our own Inner Nurturer. This experience allows us to learn firsthand the value and importance of self-love and self-care. It is also a very effective way to relax.

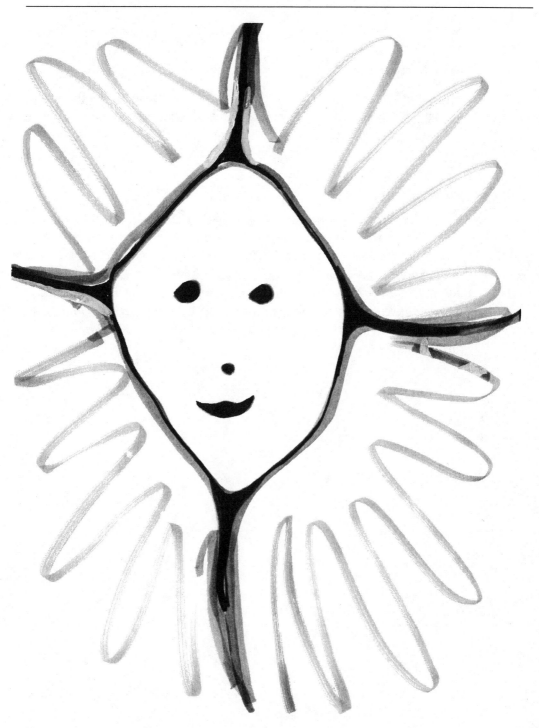

DIALOGUE WITH INNER NURTURER

Dear Nurturing Being,

You came out of the rose I was drawing. You seem so light, tender and loving, yet firm and strong. Who are you and what message do you have for me?

Oh Dear One,

I am your very soul and reflection of who you really are. I live in the heart of the flower where all the petals meet. I am the Flower Prince. Live your life like I am—soft and gentle—vulnerable and truly loving and compassionate. But your stem or core is strong, agile and ready for action like a warrior. Obedience and surrender is your armor. Courage is your shield, duty your bow, and right action your arrow. You fight so that you can enjoy the beauty you see in all the flowers. Remember, I am always with you.

NURTURING PARENT/VULNERABLE CHILD

Sit quietly for a moment. Think about the part of your personality that is like a Nurturing Parent: caring for people, animals, plants, and the environment. Then think about the part that is like a Vulnerable Child. This is the sensitive childlike part that feels sad, hurt, confused, awkward, lonely, and needs love and attention.

With your non-dominant hand, draw a picture of the Nurturing Parent and the Vulnerable Child together.

Now, take two different colored markers and write out a conversation between the Nurturing Parent and the Vulnerable Child. Let the Nurturing Parent write with your dominant hand and your Inner Child with your non-dominant hand. Let the Nurturing Parent ask the Child how it feels and what it needs today. Then, let the Nurturing Parent tell specifically how it will meet the Inner Child's needs.

Benefits: Most of us are in the unconscious habit of repressing our Inner Child. Through others' standards we learn to judge the feelings of our Child Self as right or wrong, good or bad, weak or strong. This leads to guilt for simply having these feelings. Whether externally imposed, or self-imposed, guilt feelings lead to more repression of emotions. Repressing feelings can lead to weight gain and other physical and emotional problems. In this exercise, you bring the Child's needs out of hiding, put them on paper, and look at them for what they truly are: feelings. This drawing and dialogue allows the Hidden Child to speak up and make you aware of its own wants and needs.

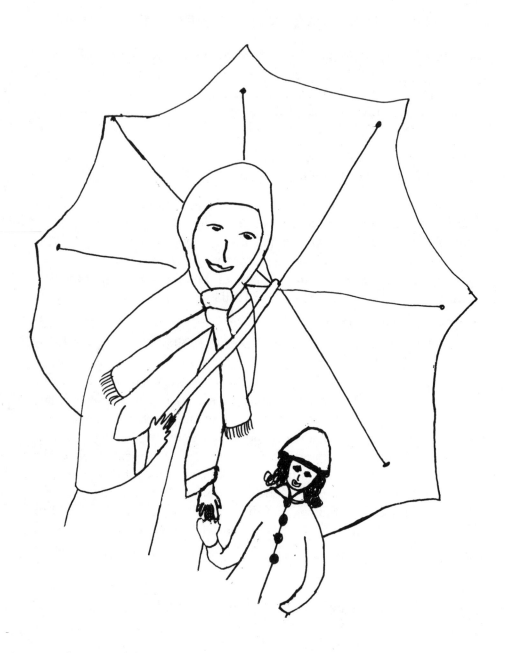

NURTURING PARENT AND VULNERABLE CHILD

NURTURING PARENT/VULNERABLE CHILD DIALOGUE

NP: I am your protector. How are you feeling today?

VC: *I am feeling fine. Just keep me warm and don't let go of my hand.*

NP: I know. It's cold out here. I'll keep the umbrella up until it stops raining. Is there anything else you need to be happy?

VC: *Hot chocolate next to the fire. And please read me a story.*

NURTURING ALL OF ME

What do you do to nurture the physical, emotional, mental, and spiritual aspects of yourself? Draw a picture of the people, places, things, and activities in your life that nurture you. As you draw each item, allow yourself to re-experience the pleasure it brings you. Display your picture as a reminder of things to do or experience.

Every day, do something to nurture and develop each of these four areas of your life. Write out a weekly list with a plan of what you intend to do for yourself. Write down the activities with your non-dominant hand. At the end of the week, review the list to see how you did.

Benefits: This is a method of observing and expressing the various aspects of your being and developing your whole self. As each part of you is getting positive attention and reinforcement, this technique can help you stay balanced. If you are having problems in any particular area, this will give you extra opportunities to express and develop yourself.

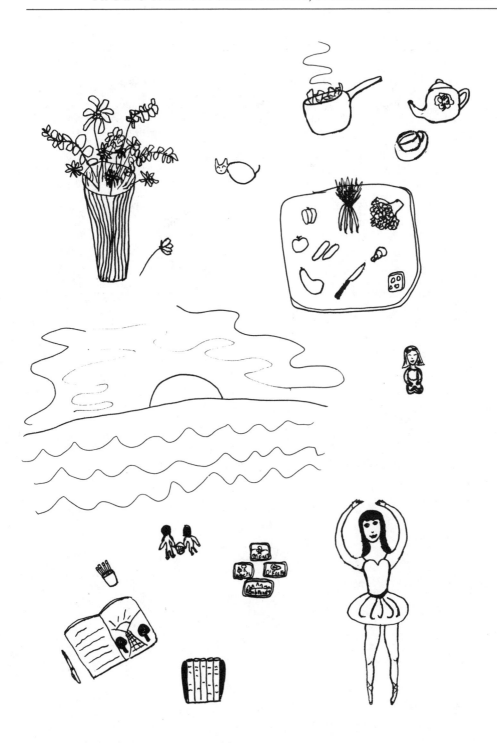

Monday	Tuesday	Wednesday	Thursday	Friday	Saturday	Sunday
Yoga/ Meditation	Yoga/ Meditation	Yoga/ Meditation	Yoga/ Meditation	Yoga/ Meditation	Yoga Class	Group Meditation
Work in Garden	Read	Flower-Arranging	Meet friend at at Cafe	Work in Garden	Lunch or Tea with Friend	Brunch with Friends
Visit Kitties Next Door	Write & Draw in Journal	Walk on Beach at Sunset	Read & Write	Read	Art Class	Walk in Park or Woods
Fix Special Dinner for Friends	Group Meditation	Read	Yoga Class	Art Opening & Dinner Out with Friends	Movie	Read Talk to Friends Long Distance

BRINGING JOY INTO MY LIFE

Draw a circle in the middle of a page and write the word "JOY" in the center. Radiating out from the circle, write down all the things that bring you joy. Draw lines connecting each item to the circle (see example).

Now, write a sentence about each "joyful" item, stating how you will further incorporate it into your present life.

Put the illustration and list up in your environment where you can look at it frequently. Commit yourself to bringing each aspect of joy into your daily life. Reread this list out loud daily as an affirmation to reinforce your goals and actions.

Benefits: This exercise is designed to develop a habit of focusing on the people, places, and activities which bring joy to your life. By identifying these joyful elements, you can integrate them into your life to create more fulfillment. When your life is filled with joy, there is less room for self-judgment and negative attitudes.

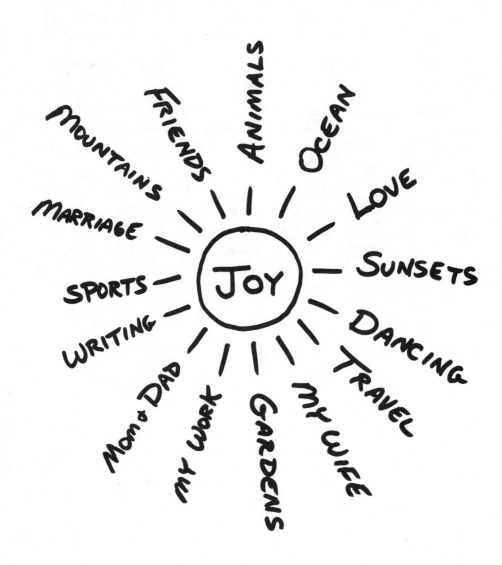

PLEASURE WALK

Do you remember the pure joy of walking to your friends' houses when you were a kid and did not have so many concerns and schedules to follow? Take a moment to think of current activities in your life which take place within reasonable walking distance of your home. Then, think of ways you can walk to these activities without having to use your car or public transportation. You may want to create special walks around your neighborhood or in parks or other natural areas.

Write a list of the places and activities to which you would like to walk to, as well as how you plan to do it. For example, you can walk to the cafe or bakery by taking the scenic route through the park.

Benefits: Walking is one of the best forms of physical exercise and can be mentally and emotionally therapeutic as well. We tend to walk a lot as kids, but begin to stop in our later teen and adult years when we discover cars. We can retrain ourselves to remember the joys of walking with a bounce in our step and a light heart. Walking for its own sake can be very nurturing.

Walk to: Museum   Printer   Restaurant
              Food Stores   Post Office   Movie Theater
              Bank   Cleaners   Photo Center

Walk to museum and afterwards stop off at the food store, bank, and printer.

Walk to beach and afterwards stop off at post office, cleaners, and deli on way home.

Walk to cafe for brunch and then down boardwalk for shopping. Go to photo center on way home.

Walk to cliffs above beach. Stop by P.O. Box and restaurant before walking home.

Walk to movie taking the scenic route through rose garden and cliffs above beach. Stop at store on way home.

PLAYTIME: FOR THE YOUNG AT HEART

Sit quietly and recall some of the things you really had fun doing when you were a kid. Make a list of these with your non-dominant hand.

As you read what you wrote, recapture the feelings of joy evoked by these memories. What can you do in your life now to recreate those feelings of simple childlike fun and joy? How can you express that playful spirit in your life? You might toss a frisbee, play with a dog or cat, ride a bike, play with crayons, paints, or clay.

You might find a friend who is willing to play a "competitive" sport with you without keeping score. Play simply for the exercise and fun of it. You might play catch with a softball, hit tennis balls, shoot baskets, or play badminton or ping pong without worrying about winning or losing.

Find a friend and a playground where you can be kids for awhile. Try the swings, slide, and jungle gym. Better yet, throw a party for the "young at heart" and hold it in a park, playground, or at a beach. Take jump ropes, squirt guns, bubble-blowing hoops, and any other toys you can think of.

Benefits: We never outgrow our need for play. Although we often associate playing with childhood games or competitive sports, the ability to play is part of being young at heart, healthy, and alive. This activity helps you to rekindle the fun you had playing when you were a kid. It gets you in touch with your natural spontaneity and creativity.

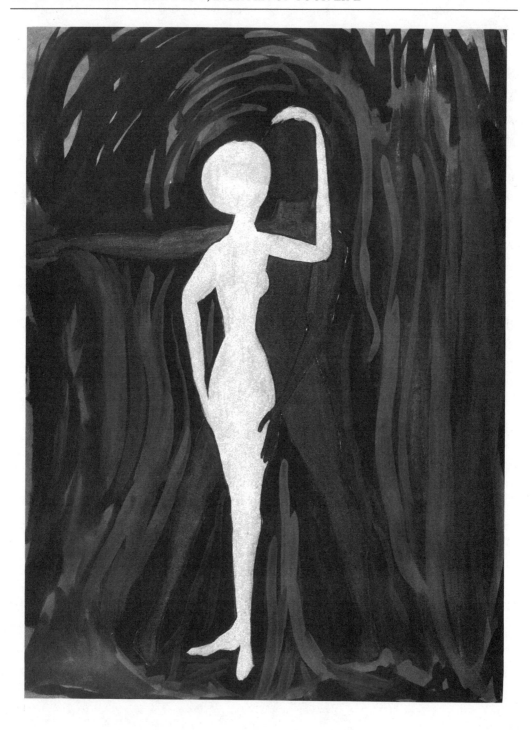

CHAPTER FIVE

Relationships That Feed the Soul

I celebrate Myself,
And what I assume you shall assume,
For every atom belonging to me as good belongs to you.

—Walt Whitman

Our relationship with ourselves and with our bodies is mirrored in our relationships with others. If we have maintained a negative body image, this will most likely show up as a negative issue somewhere in our relationships. Feelings of low self-esteem cast shadows in our minds about our attractiveness in the eyes of others. Feeling unattractive is connected to the belief that we do not deserve love. In this frame of mind we are often unable to receive love from others, even when it is offered. In extreme cases of low self-esteem, we may actually think that we deserve abuse. These feelings inevitably lead to emotional isolation and prevent us from asking for help and support.

If we go into a relationship feeling unattractive and unlovable—whether it be a friendship, partnership, or marriage—it is easy to slip into jealousy, envy, and insecurity. This is especially true in marriage and love relationships where there is physical intimacy. People who constantly ask themselves, "Who could love this body?" will mistrust anyone else's attraction to them. It will be difficult for them to receive genuine, heartfelt expressions of love from their partner, and they may live in constant fear of betrayal, even when it is unwarranted. They may even be drawn into a relationships where betrayal is inevitable, thereby proving: "I am unattractive. I am not lovable enough."

A negative body image can lead to a desperate need for approval from others. The script goes something like this: "I don't like my body, but if someone else does, then I guess I'm okay (for now)." Of course when the other person leaves, these feelings of attractiveness leave with them. This pattern can lead to an addiction to sex, romance, or relationships in which we expect others to do our self-esteem work for us. When the other person fails to bolster our feelings of attractiveness and lovableness, we tend to get angry, hurt, or withdrawn.

Other forms of relationship addiction resulting from poor body image and a sense of being unlovable are sexual and relationship anorexia. This is an avoidance of intimate relationships, and is referred to clinically as "acting in." In this case, the individual uses poor body image (and the consequent body language) to keep people away. The need for insulation and isolation may be caused by unhealed trauma, such as early physical or sexual abuse.* Our relationships begin to heal as we learn to love ourselves and our bodies. In treating ourselves with compassion, tenderness and understanding, we set the stage for healthy, loving relationships with others.

In the following exercises we explore our relationships by discovering the depth of our self-acceptance and self-love. Although extra weight very often serves as extra "protection" or insulation from emotional hurt and abuse, we cannot be totally isolated from the world around us. By developing our own inner strength and creating healthy boundaries from within, we can gradually let go of the physical protection or armoring which extra weight often represents. This chapter shows you that by first creating a loving relationship with yourself and your body, you can then create loving relationships with others in your life.

---

*If that is the case, or if memories of abuse arise while doing this work, we urge you to seek professional help at once. Such issues should not be dealt with alone or in isolation.

WHO DO YOU LOVE?

Make a list of everyone you love in your life right now. Then, in a second column list the reasons why you love each individual person.

Look over your list. Think about what you give and receive from each relationship. Is there anything in these relationships that you would like to be different? Write out what you would like to change and what *you* can do to bring about that change.

Benefits: As we do inner work to Lighten Up, we often find it necessary to examine our personal relationships in order to see if they reflect and support the changes in our lives. This exercise enables you to get a clearer picture of your relationships, and to see what changes you need to make at this time.

YOU LIGHT UP MY LIFE

Write a letter to someone who brings a great deal of joy and love into your life. Tell this person what he or she has given you simply by being themselves. Thank the person for all they have brought into your life. Be specific and tell them exactly what you appreciate about them.

Benefits: By expressing gratitude we create receptivity to more blessings in our life. This letter can be kept in your journal or copied and sent to the person to whom it was written. By sending these letters you are sharing and multiplying the joy you feel.

Dear Carol,

Thank you for being yourself with me. You give me permission to be myself, to tell the truth about who I am because you do that so well. You always seem willing to share your feelings and needs with me, no matter what. When you show your sadness, confusion, happiness, anger, you make it easy for me to show all of my feelings too. I never feel judged by you. I have learned that the kind of acceptance you show towards me is what love is all about.

With much gratitude,

Your Husband

Dear Mom,

There is so much I want to thank you for that I hardly know where to begin. There are little things like taking in my cats when I moved to New York, knitting me that beautiful long cape, helping me financially—always it seems!

But there are more important things too. First of all, you are the least judgmental person I know. Secondly, you have always been optimistic and very supportive regarding me and my variety of careers. Also, I know you are concerned about all your children—but you have the ability to keep this concern in perspective to your own life and not let it ruin your own happiness.

You're also a lot of fun! And, somehow you keenly understand why I've lived so far away from home since I left for college some 18 years ago.

I think that you're a wonderful woman, and I love you very much.

Honey

RELATIONSHIPS: LIGHT AND HEAVY

List all the people in your life whose presence or memory usually evokes negative or "heavy" feelings, such as: discomfort, distrust, anger, irritation, or unworthiness. Contemplate each person for a moment. Then, next to their name write down the feelings you associate with that person.

Now, list all the people whose presence or memory normally evokes positive or "light" feelings, such as: happiness, humor, trust, love, warmth, and support. Contemplate each person for a moment. Then, after their name write down the feelings which come up when you think about them.

When you are making a decision about entering into any kind of relationship, be it personal, professional, or social, try the following meditation:

> Sit quietly. Close your eyes and picture the person you have in mind. How do you feel when you think about this person? Recall your experience of this person. What is it like being in their presence? Do you feel confident, centered, comfortable? Can you be yourself with this person? Or do you feel uneasy, confused, manipulated or intimidated? Is there a feeling of lightness about your interactions or is it an uncomfortable experience?

Benefits: This exercise is intended to help you listen to your intuitions and impressions about other people. If you are honest about your feelings towards others, you will be able to make better choices about who you draw, or allow into your life. Lightening up means unburdening yourself from relationships that do not support you. This is done by creating boundaries and setting limits out of respect for yourself and your own needs.

HEAVY

Roger:	Distrustful	Manipulated	Hurt
	Confused	Battered	Deceived
	Rejected	Harassed	Overwhelmed
	Angry	Used	Fearful
	Vulnerable	Trapped	

LIGHT

Marianne:	Accepted	Safe	Relaxed
	Loved	Nurtured	Happy
	Peaceful	Free	Supported
	Funny	Cheerful	

DOING FOR OTHERS, DOING FOR MYSELF

Make a list of the things you do for other people, such as family members, friends, co-workers, or social groups. Include the things you enjoy doing, as well as those you do begrudgingly.

Read your list over, and select one you resent doing, are bored with, or are angry at "having to do." Now, with your non-dominant hand, draw a picture of yourself doing it. In cartoon balloons or captions, write out exactly what you would like to say and do instead of carrying out that activity.

Go back to your original list and write down all the ways you can stop doing the things you really do not want to do. Create healthy compromises or alternatives (getting sick does not count!). For instance, your husband can do his own laundry, the kids can make their own breakfasts, your wife can take out the garbage, your neighbor can buy his own tools, your boss can make his own coffee, the scout troup can get a new leader, your mother-in-law can stay home every other Sunday.

Write out all the possible solutions. Choose one, then act on it.

Benefits: When doing for others brings up any resentment or ill-will, we are "putting poison in the chicken soup." Under the guise of nurturing others we are really damaging the relationship by giving with resentment. We are also harming ourselves by repressing our true feelings and not caring for ourselves enough to say, "no."

HEALTHY RELATIONSHIPS

Sometimes life feels like a battle which we have to struggle through alone—like orphaned children with no one to be there for us. The truth is that we do not have to approach life as a solitary journey. We can call upon our own support team whenever we choose. When we reach out to others we give them a gift: the opportunity to open their hearts to us and lend a helping hand.

Make a list of some key relationships in your life: relatives, loved ones, friends, co-workers, neighbors.

Look at your list. Which of these people do you consider part of your support team? Which ones accept you as you are, believe in you, and cheer you on to reach your goals and fulfill your dreams? Which of the people on your list are critical of you, controlling, overprotective, or abusive? Which ones are never there for you? Which ones make promises that they never deliver?

If you could change one of those relationships, how would your new picture look? Draw it and then describe in writing how you would like the relationship to be. Use your non-dominant hand. You can repeat this exercise periodically to see if any changes in the relationship have come about. This can be done with as many relationships as you like.

Benefits: Healthy relationships are characterized by mutual support, and by give and take in both directions. Many who grew up in dysfunctional families did not have models for healthy relationships. Abusive or absentee parents or caregivers cannot teach children about mutual support. In this exercise you are encouraged to examine the quality of your relationships and envision new ways of relating.

FACE TO FACE

Stand in front of a mirror. Gently, with love, look at your face. Scan your face from your hairline to your neck. What do you notice about the reflection in the mirror? Does your face look back at you with love?

Let your gaze tell your reflection in the mirror that you care about it, that you are willing to try to make it truly happy.

Write down whatever comes to mind about your face. Then, draw a picture of your face as you see it.

Reread what you have written. Are the words loving, helpful, compassionate? Or are the words hateful, depressed, angry? What qualities do you see in the picture you have drawn?

Now, think about how you would like to feel about your face. Write a paragraph about how you can make this a reality.

Benefits: This exercise gets you directly in touch with how you really feel about your face and your body. It can help mend the gap between the face you show to the world, and your true inner feelings.

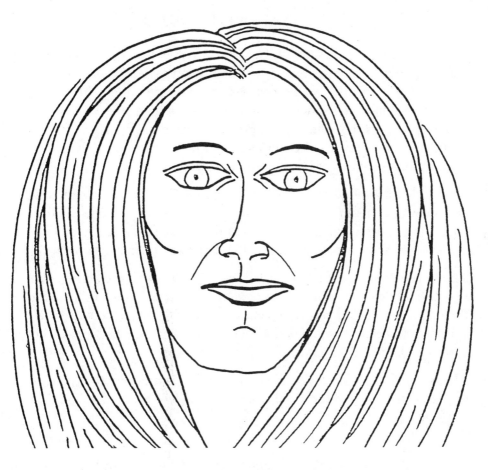

MY FACE

Sometimes I am amazed at how dumb that face can look. I feel as if I've been through wars and yet it doesn't seem to show on my face at all. In a way that's a comfort. I can start fresh. In a way it's false, though. It's a convenient shield against the world.

I would prefer to be able to say that I can believe my face—that it's honest and true. I want it to show love and wisdom. I have complete faith, however, that "years" will give me that maturity. I just wish that "years" would hold off on the gray hair. . . .

I plan to try to concentrate on not being phony and to try to be free to laugh a lot. The laughter I seek will surely give character to a face—no need to seek tears.

THE HE AND SHE INSIDE ME

The famous Swiss psychologist, C. G. Jung, recognized that there were male and female energies present in the human psyche. He referred to them as the anima (the inner female in a man) and animus (the inner male in a woman). The ancient Chinese philosophers referred to these two energies as yin (feminine, receptive) and yang (male, active). In this exercise we are going to discover our inner male and inner female, and explore the dynamics between these two forces.

Sit quietly for a moment. Close your eyes and visualize two characters, one male and one female. Pretend that these two characters live within you. Allow your imagination to express these two characters in any figures, colors, shapes, or sizes you wish. Give each character a name.

Then, allow these characters to have a conversation with each other. Use two different colored markers, one for the female character and one for the male character. If you are a woman, allow the "male" to write with your non-dominant hand. If you are a man, let your "female" speak with your non-dominant hand.

After completing your dialogue you may want to draw another picture of the inner male and female showing the way you would *like* them to relate to each other.

Benefits: Discovering the male and female energies in our psyche can help us uncover attitudes and beliefs that block and sabotage our relationships. Once revealed, we can begin to heal ourselves and become more whole. Then, we are more capable of having a healthy intimate relationship with another.

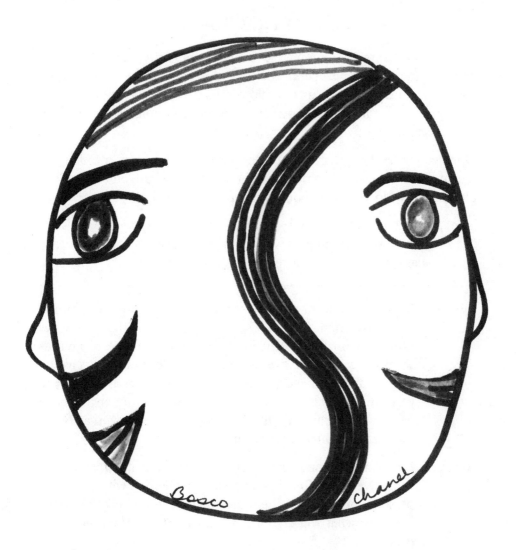

Masculine: My name is Bosco. I am tall, dark and handsome. I do all the things a man should—but I also contain tenderness and emotion for the woman. I am the dark and light together, although my role is to be strong – courageous – protective – honest – smart and negotiate for things in life that make life good and comfortable for me and my woman.

Feminine: I am Chanel. I like all things soft and feminine – flowers – candlelight dinners – gifts – surprises – kitty cats – clothes – travel – gardens – food – art – beautiful surroundings – sunsets – walks in nature – and long dark sensual nights with my man.

LIKE ATTRACTS LIKE

Think about the perfect intimate love relationship for you. Picture it and imagine how you would feel in this relationship. What qualities would you experience? What feelings would you have for the other person? Sit very quietly for a moment, close your eyes and contemplate this perfect relationship.

Open your eyes. Draw a picture of this perfect relationship in which you feel loved and are loved. Write a paragraph about what you drew in the picture. How do you feel about yourself and your life?

Then, write a second paragraph about how you can experience the state of being which you pictured above, right now. What can you specifically do to make this loving state a reality in your life?

Benefits: Most people want a loving relationship because they think it will make them happy. They focus on what they want the other person to be. But in looking for someone to give us what we don't have, we become dependent on others as the suppliers of our needs. This is giving our power away. In contrast, this exercise helps us develop our own inner power so we can attract another like being. Become what you are looking for and you will attract it.

Note: If you are in a long-term or on-going relationship, this exercise can be very helpful. When you are dissatisfied with the other person, you can shift the focus to yourself and take responsibility for *what you are*, rather than *what you think he or she is or is not.*

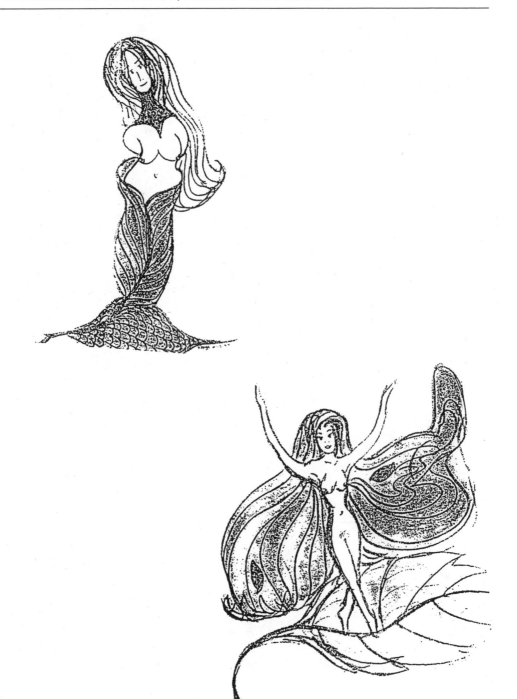

CHAPTER SIX

Emerging from the Cocoon: Finding Your Light Body

If the doors of perception were cleansed, everything would appear as it is, infinite.

For man has closed himself up, till he sees all things through the narrow chinks of his cavern.

—William Blake

As a culture we have come to view our bodies with fear and suspicion. Religion tells us that the body is sinful, and its impulses and feelings cannot be trusted. We are reminded of the temptations and weaknesses of the flesh. For thousands of years philosophers have carefully separated the soul from the body. Scientists have described the body as a "machine" to be ruled by the dictates of the mind. The result has been that the mind has become a petty dictator over the body, and our bodies have suffered the consequences.

We have also come to believe in the "ideal" body which everyone strives for. However, we tend to forget that over the centuries cultures have always differed in their ideas about the most desirable and perfect human form. The "ideal form" has varied from the classical proportions of the ancient Greeks to the round, sensuous bodies as seen in Renaissance art. Today, we have the thin but athletic "Hollywood" body of America in the 1980's. These are all simply concepts projected upon the human body.

In fact, our human body is not unlike the alien light beings in the movie *Cocoon,* who were encased in their own mysterious cocoons. As humans,

123

we exist in our own protective shell, superimposed over our natural body. These shells are molded and held together by our own unique psychological and emotional armoring. Their density insulates and protects us from the physical and emotional demands of our environment, allowing us to live "safely" in the world.

Although the creation of our "cocoon" began in childhood, it is sustained in adulthood by our beliefs about health, eating, nourishment, our body, and our self. Many of these beliefs may be outworn and destructive to our physical and emotional states. They may sound something like this: "Eating makes me fat," "Overweight runs in my family," "I gain weight when I stop smoking," "People get fat as they get older," "I have to diet and exercise in order to be thin," "Stress causes me to eat more."

As we begin to love ourselves and develop healthier attitudes, we may also experience corresponding changes in the structure or design of our cocoon. The body will often reorganize and reshape itself into a more flexible, fluid, and lighter form. This process of transformation can be enhanced through the regenerating powers of deep relaxation and natural breathing.

We can use our own natural breathing to help us descend to that profound revitalizing state we experience in deep sleep. Our breath is the key: it is the connecting link between mind and body. As the breathing rhythm slows and becomes more balanced, the mind and body automatically relax, and our awareness of the body increases. It is this energized and relaxed state of awareness that is the foundation and starting point for true change and healing.

As we enter deep relaxation, there is a remarkable shift in our bodily awareness: from a feeling of heaviness to a feeling of lightness, from feeling low energy to feeling high energy, and from feeling "disconnected" to experiencing a balanced and integrated wholeness. In this state we can discover the perfect design of our human body as we were meant to experience it, *from the inside out*. This perfect body can be experienced through relaxation, movement awareness, meditation, and peak physical experiences. We refer to it as our Light Body.

In this chapter you will learn to recognize and change the beliefs which you have held about your body. You will discover your own Light Body through drawings, dialogues, mirror work, meditations, and movement. As you shed your outworn beliefs, like an old suit of clothes, you will be stepping out of a cocoon to reveal the naturally vibrant Light Body which has been waiting all along to emerge.

I HEARD IT THROUGH THE GRAPEVINE

Write down all the "sayings" you have heard in relation to weight, bodies, food, etc. Include things people have warned you about or predicted for you.

After writing down as many sayings as you can think of, place a star next to every "saying," warning, or prediction that you have personally used or believed.

Next, rewrite each negative into a "positive reality."

Benefits: Unfortunately, most of us believed the sayings and warnings or predictions given to us throughout the years. Because we believed them, we also became the manifestation of those harmless sayings. Now, you are living for "you," and can believe what you choose to believe. This is the perfect time to turn all the sayings and warnings around to work for you, and make all the predictions healthy ones.

OLD SAYINGS ABOUT FOOD AND WEIGHT

If you are fat as a child, you will always be fat.
I have the same weight problem as my mother.
If you don't exercise, your muscles will turn to flab.
You have to follow a strict diet to lose weight.
You need to eat a big breakfast to make it through the day.
If you eat too much, you'll get sick.
You have to eat or you'll get sick.
Don't eat those cookies or you'll spoil your appetite.
If you eat sweets, you will ruin your teeth.
A moment on the lips, a month on the hips.

POSITIVE REWRITES

If I am fat as a child, I can be slender as an adult.
Some people in my family had problems with their weight.
If I don't exercise, I won't get flabby.
I can lose weight without dieting.
I only need a light breakfast to be healthy.
If I eat too much, I will try not to next time.
I eat when I am hungry.
If I eat a few cookies, my appetite will not be affected.
If I brush my teeth, a few sweets won't bother me.
A moment on the lips, forever thin hips.

MY BODY IS . . .

Write the word "Body" in the center of the page. Draw a circle around it.

Pick a colored marker and, around the circle, write all your negative thoughts about your body.

Pick another color and, around the circle, write all your positive thoughts about your body.

Make a list of all your negative thoughts about your body. Change each one, in writing, to a positive thought.

If there is resistance to changing a negative belief to a positive, simply keep writing the positive over and over until *the writing of it* feels comfortable to you.

Benefits: In order to change our bodies, we must change the negative beliefs we have about our bodies. This exercise is an important step in this process, as you are given an opportunity to turn negative beliefs and conditions into positive beliefs and blessings that can work for you.

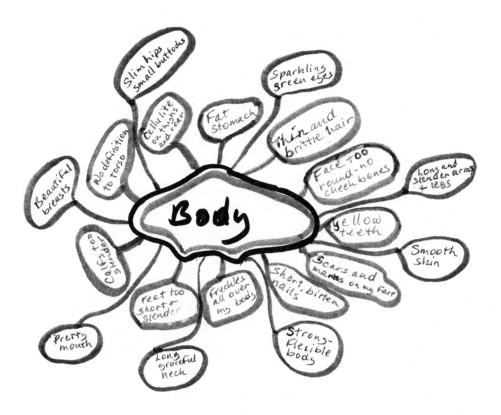

NEGATIVE	POSITIVE
Cellulite on thighs and rear.	I am letting go of the anger I store in my thighs & rear.
Fat stomach	I am strengthening my lower back & abdominal muscles to better hold my stomach and to balance my well-toned buttocks.
Thin and brittle hair	My hair is getting stronger, thicker and more lustrous.
Scars and marks on my face	My face is truth and reflects the inner beauty and wisdom of a fully-lived life.
Short bitten nails	My hands have full expression and energy to do all the great things they have to do.
Undefined torso	My torso works hard to uphold my chest & upper body & graciously encases my spine.
Yellow teeth	My teeth never waiver in their constant daily chewing of the nourishing foods I take in my body.

DIALOGUE WITH A HEAVYWEIGHT

Draw a picture of someone whose body is "heavy" and unattractive to you.

Have a written conversation with the person in that picture. Let the heavy person write with your non-dominant hand. Ask why they look the way they do and how it feels to be in their body.

Now, ask the person in the picture to draw their Light Body—their naturally healthy, vibrant body. Have a written conversation with their Light Body, allowing it to write with your non-dominant hand. Ask how it feels to live in a Light Body, and how it feels to be trapped inside a heavy or unattractive body.

Benefits: This exercise helps us to stop identifying with an unattractive self that we criticize and judge, and to see it as a "character" we have created in our mind. By getting to know it and how it feels, we can develop understanding and compassion. It also lets us see beneath the surface to discover the natural Light Body hidden in our current physical form.

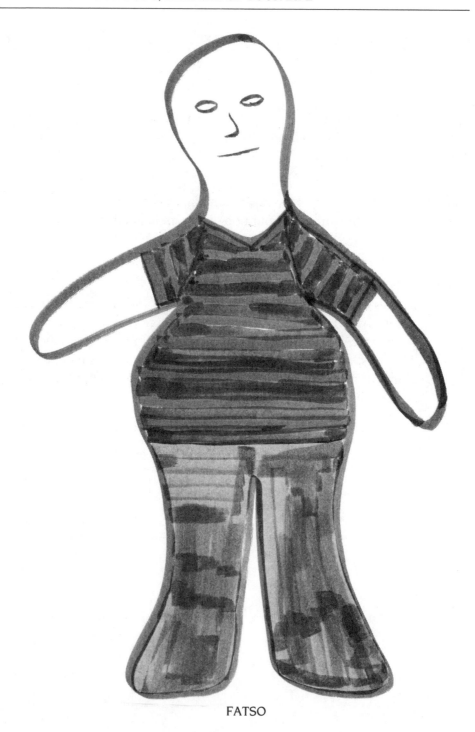

FATSO

DIALOGUE WITH FATSO

Hi! Who are you?

I'm Fatso.

How are you feeling?

Okay, I guess. It's so hard to move around in this big body. It feels like I'm wearing a football uniform made of lead. I feel so weighted down.

What happened? Why are you walking around in such a heavy body?

I dunno. Ate too much, I guess. I was never too good at sports & everybody made fun of me. Nobody wanted me on their team. So I stopped playing with the kids and stayed home. My mom is a good cook & gave me plenty to eat cause I'm so good in school. I got to eat all I want when I made an A.

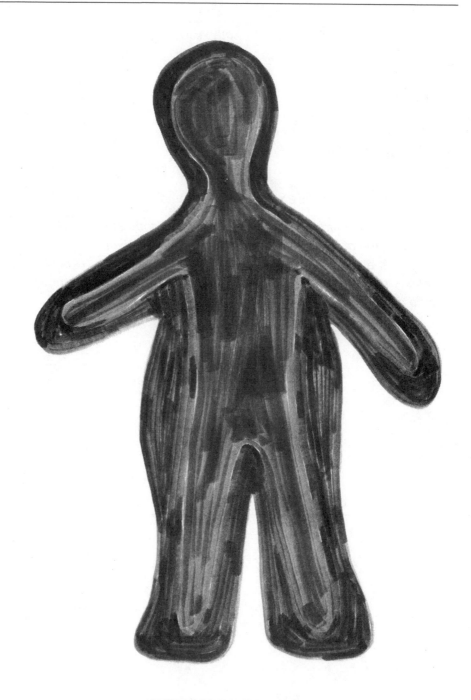

LIGHT BODY INSIDE FATSO

DIALOGUE WITH LIGHT BODY

Hi! Who are you?

The Light Body.

How do you feel?

Wonderful. I am pure energy. So light and vibrant. Everything feels so effortless.

How does it feel to be trapped inside of Fatso's body?

Real boring. Fatso carries around so much extra baggage that he can't even feel me. It feels like trying to swim against the current. It takes so much effort to do anything.

Sometimes I call him "Mr. Molasses." His body doesn't work. If he knew about me, it would be so easy for him. But he doesn't have a clue. One of these days though, I'm gonna be free! I want to laugh and dance and sing again!

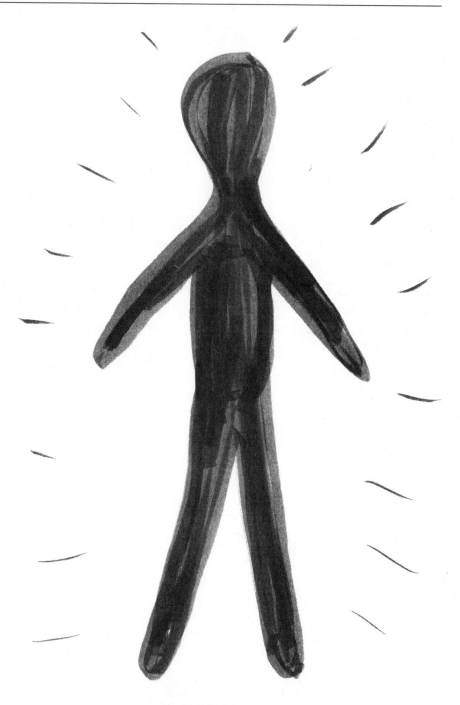

LIGHT BODY

REFLECTIONS OF LOVE

Stand in front of a full-length mirror in as little clothing as possible. Quietly and calmly gaze at your body from head to toe. Examine your reflection from the front, sides, and back.

As you look at your reflection, notice if there is anything about your body that you dislike. Be aware of any critical thoughts or judgments which arise in your mind. As critical thoughts arise, replace them with a feeling of love and compassion for your body. Thank your body for how it has served you in your life. How does it feel to look at your body without judgment?

As you continue to look at yourself in the mirror, compliment yourself out loud or in your mind, focusing on the positive qualities you see in your reflection. Allow the feelings of love and appreciation for your body to grow. Now, see if your body feels any different than it did at the beginning of this exercise. Does it appear any different to your eyes?

Benefits: The picture of our bodies which we carry in our mind can be corrected with self-love and compassion. This exercise is very important because it shows you where your dissatisfaction is coming from—your own attitude. You can also learn what you need to work on to alter those old critical pictures and change your body to match your new beliefs and images.

TREE OF LIGHT MEDITATION

With your eyes closed, imagine yourself as a tree growing out of the ground. Your roots are energy coming up from the earth through your feet. Visualize this energy as light and let it circulate slowly through your entire being, filling and expanding each area of your body. If there are any areas of tension, stress, or pain, let the light dissolve the darkness or discomfort in those areas. You can help the process by directing your breath energy to those distressed areas and affirming, "My (body part) is relaxed." Let yourself feel the tingling sensation all over that comes with complete relaxation and well-being. Imagine a white light around your body, emanating from within. Feel the protection and comfort that this white light gives you.

Benefits: Here we are using visualization, sense perception, and affirmation to create a state of relaxation and wellness for the body. It is especially helpful in times of stress, low energy, or fatigue. This meditation can be calming and rejuvenating at the same time, bringing about an even and natural flow of energy throughout your body.

WALKING IN YOUR LIGHT BODY

Pretend you are in the very best possible physical condition—healthy, happy, and very pleased with your weight and appearance. You are on top of the world and everything is going your way.

Stand up and walk around the room as if everything in your life is just the way you want it. You might want to select some of your favorite uplifting or inspirational music, and walk or move to the rhythm of the sound.

Remember, you are in great shape and look fabulous, so walk that way! Enjoy it! Notice how you are walking. How does your body feel when you walk this way? Is there any difference between this experience and your normal walk? Does it feel lighter and more energetic? Keep walking and note all the differences and similarities.

When you are ready, write down how you feel about the Light Body Walk. Let the words come spontaneously. You may want to draw a picture of how it felt to walk in your Light Body.

Benefits: Imagining the pleasant physical experience of walking in our Light Body reinforces our motivation to change, and helps make it a tangible reality to us. The more we exerience the physical actions and feelings associated with our own Light Body, the more we are able to "embody" it.

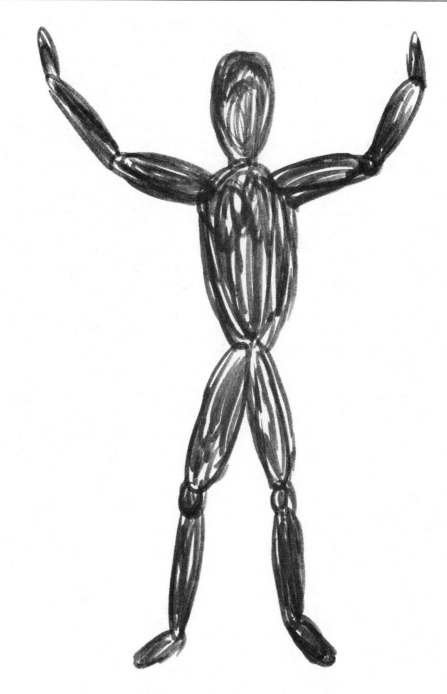

WALKING IN MY LIGHT BODY

DISCOVERING YOUR LIGHT BODY: SKIPPING

Think about how joyful and carefree children look when they are skipping. Can you remember how it felt?

Find a place where you feel safe to skip: in your backyard, your living room (if large enough), a park, the playground, or the beach. Go for it! Skip to your heart's content!

How do you feel while skipping? How does your body feel?

Now, using your non-dominant hand, draw a picture of how you felt as you were skipping. Write down any words or phrases which come to mind as you draw the picture.

Benefits: It is hard not to smile and feel light and happy when you are skipping. Although it may seem very unadult to be seen skipping around the neighborhood, your Inner Child loves to skip. The rhythm and grace of the movement makes you feel truly alive! Also, for those who do not like to run, this is a fun and wonderful way to get some exercise.

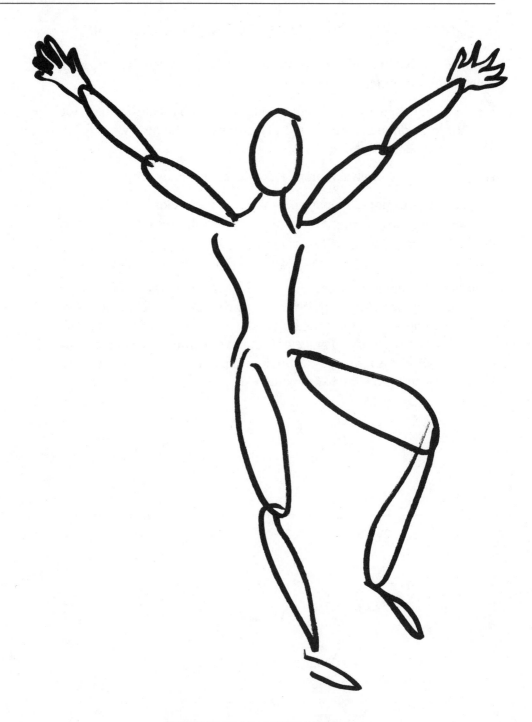

SKIPPING IN MY LIGHT BODY

DANCING IN YOUR LIGHT BODY

Everyone has different taste in music. Some prefer classical while others like jazz, rock, or swing. Put on some music which makes your body want to move. As you start to move to the music, let your body take the lead. Forget stereotyped "dance steps" or forms of dance. Feel the music and let your body respond to it, letting the movement come from the inside out.

You can experiment with all kinds of movement: jumping, twirling, leaping, running, skipping, and turning. As you dance let your Inner Child out to play.

As you relax into moving to the music, visualize your Light Body dancing with ease and grace. "Become" your Light Body and experience freedom and joy in your dance.

Benefits: Spontaneous dance is a key to freeing up the body from stress and emotional blocks, and encouraging youthfulness and enthusiasm. When you explore movement with the curiosity and playfulness of a child, you liberate a magical source of creativity within yourself.

DRAWING OUT YOUR LIGHT BODY

Close your eyes and sit quietly for a moment. Listen to your breathing and allow your body and mind to relax.

Contemplate the experiences you have had with your Light Body in the previous exercises. Visualize how it would be to live in this body all the time. See yourself moving about freely and gracefully in everyday activities. Notice how you feel being radiant, alive, and self-assured.

Now, using your non-dominant hand, draw a picture of your Light Body. Use as many colors as you like.

Allow the picture of your Light Body to speak, expressing how it feels in words and phrases. Use the first person present tense. For instance, "I radiate health and vitality." You can write these words and phrases around the picture.

Display this picture in your environment where you can see it regularly. Repeatedly viewing the picture of your Light Body serves as a visual reminder of the way you would like to live in your body all the time. Use the written phrases as verbal affirmations. Repeat them mentally throughout the day, and at the same time, recall the drawing of your Light Body.

Benefits: Through verbal and visual affirmations, this activity helps you to integrate the experience of your Light Body into your everyday life.

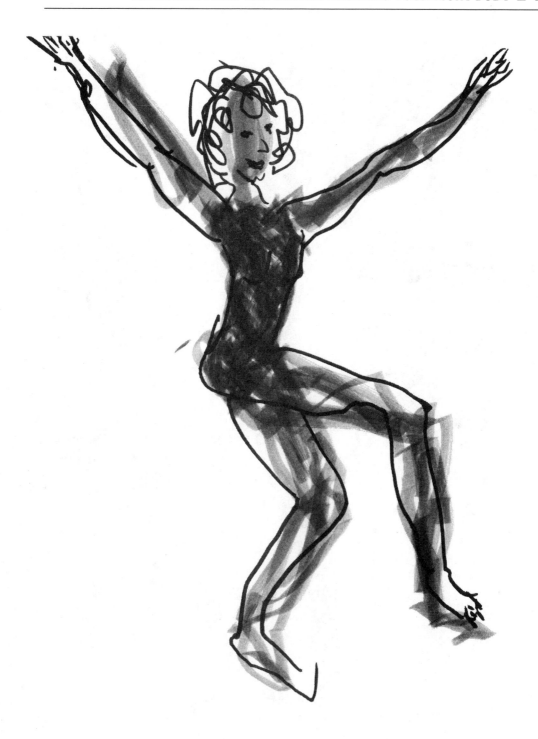

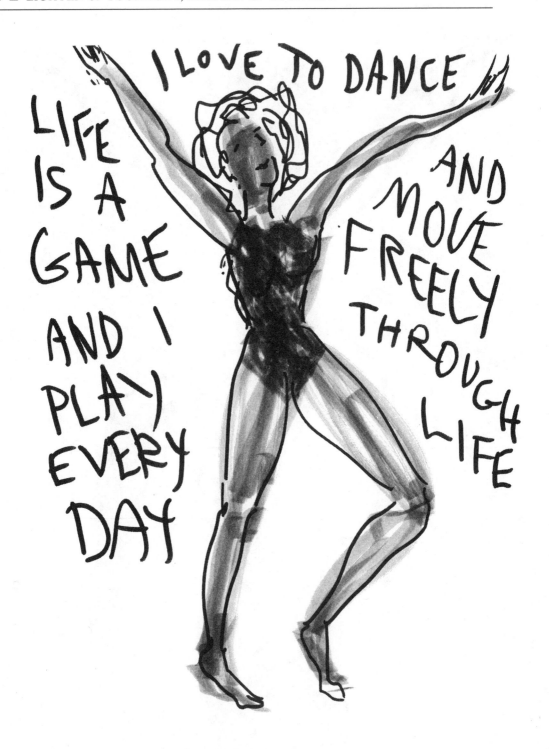

Walk in the rhythm of life;
Your limbs will not tire.
Sing with the rhythm of life;
Your voice will gain sweetness.
Dance in the rhythm of life;
Your feet will not touch the ground.
Breathe in rhythm.
Think in rhythm.
Sing in rhythm.
Dance in rhythm.
Let rhythm be your life.

Paramananda

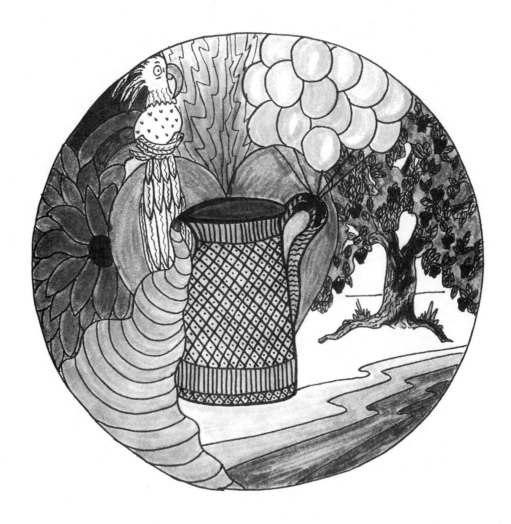

CHAPTER SEVEN

Your Life as a Work of Art

If you can dream it, you can do it.

—Walt Disney

We have an unlimited source of creativity within us at all times. It is this creativity which makes us human, enabling us to change and grow. By tapping into this creativity, we can fashion our lives according to our own vision, instead of acting out borrowed dreams. For example, many people find themselves in unsatisfying careers or unhappy marriages. In many cases, the initial choice was motivated by a need for security or approval from parents or peers. Such choices do not spring from an inner knowing, but from external pressures to conform or please. Under these circumstances the job or relationship lacks heart. It becomes dry and hollow, a matter of drudgery or duty to be endured rather than enjoyed.

A life lived creatively, on the other hand, is like a work of art in progress. It unfolds from within, responding to its own unique impulses and rhythm. A life lived creatively is like no other life—it does not imitate others but is authentic and true to itself. Like a great artist, such a person has a character and style all their own. They do not automatically accept "the way things have always been," but question commonly held beliefs. Such a person understands that beliefs shape our bodies and our lives, and they are willing to redesign their beliefs in order to live more fully, and to express the vision in their heart.

In this chapter you will learn how to apply your innate creativity to your own life. You are the raw material and you are also the artist. However, in order to give birth to "the new you," it is necessary to do some house-cleaning and get rid of old habits and beliefs. For this task you will be provided tools for creatively approaching everyday problems, and using them as a medium for your personal growth.

The word "problem" usually triggers a feeling of anxiety in people. It is associated with difficulty, fear, confusion, and pain. Problems are seen as something to be gotten rid of as soon as possible. Problems mean trouble. However, a creative way of approaching problems is to see them as friends or allies bearing gifts, rather than enemies to be avoided.

In this chapter you learn how to stop procrastinating and running away from your problems. In fact, you will be able to turn and face them, and literally talk with them. Whether you have issues regarding your health, body image, career, or relationships, you can learn how to discover the solution within the problem itself. Engaging in this kind of creative problem-solving liberates a tremendous amount of energy for the task of reshaping your health and your life the way you want it. It also generates the necessary enthusiasm for following through on your visions, especially when the going gets rough.

As you begin expressing your dreams and visions on paper, you will be singing your "heartsong." As you allow yourself to play with possibilities, you will discover the power of your inner strength and wisdom. Through the guidance of your Inner Self or Higher Power, you will be shown how to live creatively—at home in your Light Body.

CLEANING UP YOUR LIFE

Contemplate the areas of your life which feel messy, cluttered, or unresolved. In what ways are you disorganized? Where do you procrastinate? What do you resist completing?

Now, picture in your mind a fabulous "Cleaning Brigade" which you have hired to help you clean up your life. This brigade consists of experts in exactly the areas where you need help. The team comes with all of the necessary equipment they need to do the job.

Select one area of your life which needs cleaning up or repair. It might be your closets or desk, bank account, career, relationships, health, or your self-esteem. Now, draw a picture of the cleaning person who is best equipped to help you with this challenge. In the picture show how this person goes full steam ahead to clean up the mess. Be sure to include yourself in the picture. You may want to have a written dialogue in which you thank the cleaning person for a job well done. Allow the cleaning person to write with your non-dominant hand.

Now, draw a picture of how this area of your life looks now that it is all cleaned up. You may want to put this picture up in your environment as a reminder of the way you would like things to be.

Benefits: Periodic cleansing is important in all aspects of our lives. By recognizing your resistance to dealing with everyday problems and then creating someone to help you, you access your own inner power. This exercise puts you in touch with the "action" part of yourself that knows how to get things done.

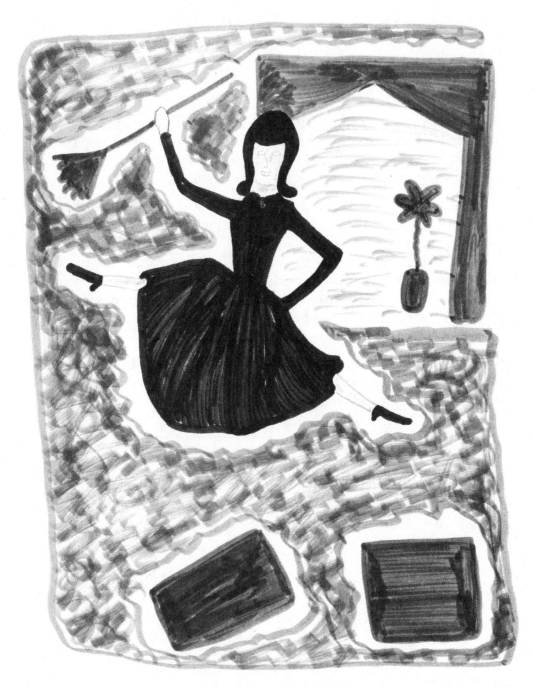

MAGICAL CLEANING LADY

LETTING YOUR PROBLEMS SOLVE THEMSELVES

Sit quietly for a moment and contemplate one area of your life that feels like a problem. It could be your physical health, your career, a relationship, your financial situation, or your home environment.

Draw a picture of the problem and give it a name. Write the name as the title under the picture.

Have a written conversation with the problem in your picture. Write the following questions with your dominant hand, and let the problem respond by writing with your non-dominant hand.

> Who or what are you?
> How do you feel?
> Why do you feel that way?
> What can I do to help you?

Benefits: This exercise encourages you to seek solutions in the place you least expect to find them—inside the problem! In fact, by doing this exercise you may learn to perceive problems in a new way, seeing them as your teachers. What you once believed were problems to be eliminated as soon as possible, can now be embraced as golden opportunities for gaining insight into yourself.

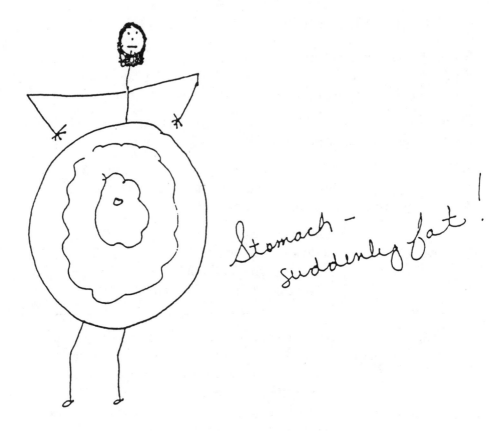

Stomach —
Suddenly fat!

DIALOGUE WITH PROBLEM

Me: Who are you?

Problem: I am your stomach.

Me: How do you feel?

Problem: Like a bowling ball.

Me: What makes you feel that way?

Problem: You do. You are tense and angry. You are blocked.

Me: What can I do to help you?

Problem: Write down exactly how you feel about John. Don't just pretend nothing happened. Write down exactly how you feel right now. Write down that you are hurt, angry, and frightened. Then write down why you feel this way. You must get clear in your own mind about all of this. When you are clear, then I suggest you call John and tell him how you feel. Don't let this go on without saying or doing anything. You worked very hard to lose all that weight—and here I am sticking out again. DO SOMETHING ABOUT IT!!!

ON TOP OF THE CLOUDS

Sit quietly for a moment. Close your eyes and listen to your natural breathing. Imagine that you are lying in a safe, firm, supporting, loving cloud. The cloud can be whatever color appeals to you—a color that feels soothing and healing.

When you are feeling safe, comfortable, and relaxed in your cloud, imagine that you are releasing the problem that you dealt with in the previous exercise. Take as long as you wish to let go of whatever is troubling you about this issue in your life. Let go of your problem and let the cloud firmly support you.

When you feel that you have let go of your problem, open your eyes and draw a picture of yourself in your safety cloud.

Then, allow the cloud to guide you. Write what it has to say using your non-dominant hand.

Benefits: In this exercise you create a supportive environment (your cloud) in which you can safely surrender your problems. The added value of allowing your supportive cloud to express itself is that it puts you in touch with your loving nurturing Inner Self.

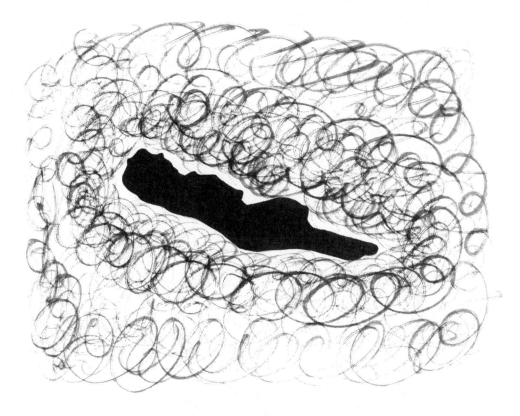

I, the cloud, though light and airy in appearance, am the essence of the mysterious simplicity of the universe. Within me is the safety of knowing that you are perfect and you are capable of doing anything you want to do. Trust yourself. Turn within to find the answers to any questions. Turn within to find me. I support you and give you safety. Turn within to find yourself.

DISCOVERING YOUR CREATIVE SELF

Take a moment to focus on your natural breathing and allow yourself to relax. Contemplate what the word "creative" means to you.

Now, draw a picture of your Creative Self using your non-dominant hand. Use whatever colors, forms, shapes, or designs you wish.

After observing the drawing carefully, ask your Creative Self, "How can you help reveal my perfect Light Body?" Allow your Creative Self to answer with your non-dominant hand.

Benefits: In this exercise you call upon your inner creativity for guidance and assistance in reclaiming your natural Light Body. Often, creative approaches to issues of weight and body image help us to break through old habits and beliefs which have blocked us in the past.

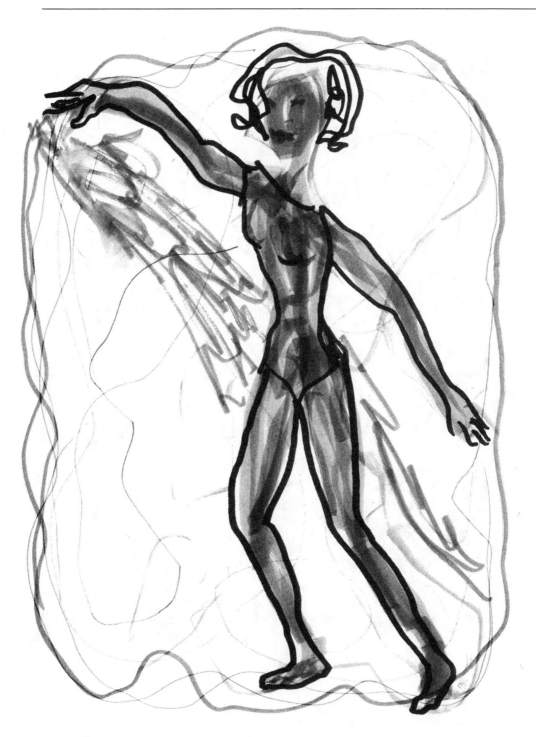

Dear Creative Self:
HOW CAN YOU HELP ME FIND
MY LIGHT BODY.
I AM YOUR LIGHT
BODY. I AM A LIGHT
BEING. BY LETTING
OUT YOUR CREATIVITY
YOU LIBERATE YOUR
TRUE SELF THE
REAL YOU. YOU
ILLUMINATE YOUR

LIFE + YOU LIGHT
UP THE WORLD. SO
LET ME OUT,
REAL-IZE YOUR
DREAMS. LIVE
YOUR DREAMS
NOW. DON'T PUT
IT OFF. REAL-IZE
YOUR SELF. LOVE
YOUR SELF.

DIALOGUE WITH CREATIVE SELF

Dear Creative Self: How can you help me find my Light Body?

Creative Self: I am your Light Body. I am a Light Being. By letting out your creativity you liberate your true self, the real you. You illuminate your life & you light up the world. So let me out, realize your dreams. Live your dreams now. Don't put it off. Realize your self. Love your self.

DRESS TO EXPRESS

Materials: Magazines with photographs, paper, scissors, glue, colored felt pens.

Contemplate the way you dress and the way it expresses who you are. What colors do you usually wear? How would you describe your style of dress—casual, sporty, artistic, ethnic, romantic, formal? Does the way you dress express who you *really* are?

Are there any changes you would like to make in your style of dress? Are there any particular colors, accessories, or other items which you have always wanted but felt were too extravagant or too different?

Now, create a collage using magazine photographs of the kinds of clothing and accessories that would give your Light Body great pleasure. Do not limit yourself in colors, textures, and designs.

When you have completed your collage, display it on the wall or on the mirror in the area where you usually get dressed. Use this picture as a visual affirmation for creating your new Light Body image.

Notice how your collage affects the way you dress. If, over a period of time, you see any changes, write about it in your journal. Better yet, have someone take photographs of you with your "new" image, and put them up next to your collage.

Benefits: The way you dress is an expression of who you are and how you feel about your body. Creating your own unique style of dress is a way of celebrating and honoring your Light Body. Many people postpone dressing the way they would really like to until they make more money, lose that "extra ten pounds," or get a promotion. Dressing to please yourself does not have to be put off any longer, and can help you create a more radiant and attractive self-image.

CREATING A NURTURING ENVIRONMENT

Materials: Magazines with photographs, paper, scissors, glue, colored felt pens.

Contemplate the kind of environment you would like to create for yourself, at home or in your work space. Visualize an environment in which your Light Body can thrive.

Make a picture using drawing and collage. Create a picture of the world you would like to create for yourself. Be sure to include yourself in the picture by drawing an image of your Light Body. Cut out words or captions in the magazines that describe what you want to create, and glue them onto your design.

Then, interview the "you" in the picture. Ask such questions as: How are you? Where are you? How did you get there? How do you feel? etc. Allow the you in the picture to answer by writing with your non-dominant hand.

Benefits: Our most wonderful fantasies can come true if we allow them to take shape in our lives, rather than just fading away in our imagination. This exercise releases your fantasy onto paper where you can see it, and recreate it over and over again. By doing the interview, you find out how you can make this fantasy come true.

LIVING IN YOUR LIGHT BODY

Materials: Magazines with photographs, paper, scissors, glue, colored felt pens.

Think about the kind of life that would nurture your Light Body: people you would like to spend time with, places you would like to visit, and things you would like to do or create in your life.

Now, create a collage with a drawing of your Light Body in the center, surrounded by photographs of the activities you want to create in your life. It may include physical activities such as sports, hiking, working out, or dancing. Your collage can also include pictures that represent loving relationships, fulfilling work, expanded social life, travel, or the arts. Display your collage in a place where you can look at it frequently. Reinforce it by recalling it in your mind as often as you can.

Focus on one thing in your collage that you really want in your life right now. Let that element of your collage speak as if the future is now and you already have what you want. What does the picture of your dream-come-true say to you? Write it out with your non-dominant hand. You can repeat this for as many elements in your collage as you would like.

Imagine that your entire collage is now a reality in your life. Write a letter to a friend describing these wonderful blessings. Tell them how you feel inside and how happy you are to be *you*, living *your* life right now. Shoot for the moon! Make this the happiest, most positive letter you have ever written.

Benefits: By creating visualizations on paper through drawing and photographic collage you can bring your dreams and fantasies more rapidly into 3-dimensional reality. When you take these images in through your eyes you are strengthening their power to influence your behavior. These pictures act as visual auto-suggestions helping you to re-program your unconscious. This is the same psychology used in advertising through billboards and magazine ads. The difference here, however, is that *you* choose the image that serves your best interests and the dream which promotes your well-being.

MEDITATING IN YOUR LIGHT BODY

Sit comfortably on the floor or in a chair. Allow your spine to be straight and slightly elongated. If you are sitting on the floor you may want to sit with a cushion under your buttocks to help support your body. If you are sitting in a chair, your legs are uncrossed with your feet flat on the floor, and your hands in your lap.

Close your eyes and become aware of your body. Are you comfortable? Does your body feel supported? Make any necessary adjustments in your posture. When your body is in a comfortable and balanced posture, begin to observe your breathing. Witness the breath coming into the body and passing out of the body.

As your breathing becomes slower, deeper, and more rhythmic, begin to *listen* to the sound of your breathing. Observe the sound as the breath comes into the body and as it goes out of the body. Continue to listen to the sound of your breathing, allowing yourself to relax more and more deeply.

Now, imagine a tiny sphere of light in the center of your heart. Feel the radiance, love, and life-giving vitality of this wondrous light. Now, ask this sphere of light to expand and spread throughout your entire body. Observe as the light slowly radiates out from your heart, filling your body. Feel the light passing down into your abdomen and legs, out into your arms, and up into your head. Allow this radiant light-energy to illuminate and nourish each and every cell in your body. Continue to bask in the splendor of this glorious light.

Benefits: Meditation can serve many functions in our lives. It is a wonderful method for relaxing and revitalizing the body and mind. By bringing about a state of inner stillness, meditation allows us to cultivate a profound inner awareness. Through this awareness we are more able to listen to the sensations and signals from our bodies. Most important, meditation allows us to listen to the messages and guidance arising from within.

DRAWING ON YOUR INNER WISDOM

Sit quietly for a moment and focus on your natural breathing. Allow your sense of relaxation to gradually deepen.

Contemplate the timeless wisdom which dwells within you. Living in each and every cell of your body, it is always there to guide you. Thank it for how it has served you unceasingly in your life, regardless of whether you were aware of it or not, or listened to any of its messages. Promise to honor your Inner Wisdom and to be more receptive to its love and guidance in your life, *starting today.*

Now, allow your Inner Wisdom to assume a form in your mind. What does it look like? It may be a wise old man, a wise old woman, or a spiritual guide. It can appear as anything which is inspiring and meaningful for you.

Draw a picture of your Inner Wisdom, however you imagine it to be. Then, write out a conversation between you and your Inner Wisdom. You write with your dominant hand and your Inner Wisdom with your non-dominant hand. Ask your Inner Wisdom for help, advice, and assistance in your journey to Lighten Up Your Body and Lighten Up Your Life.

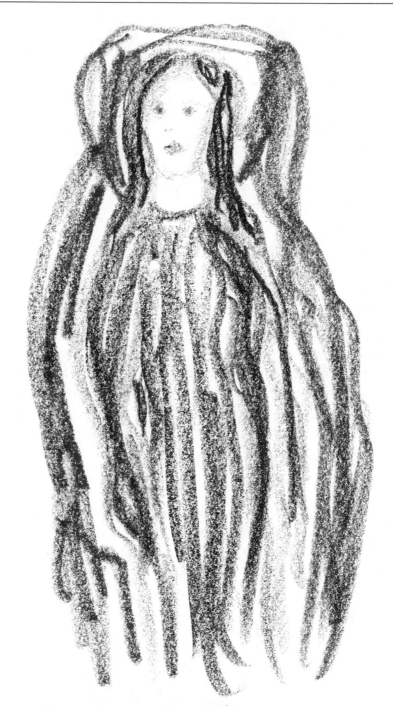

INNER GUIDE

DIALOGUE WITH INNER GUIDE

Dear Inner Guide: Please guide me in Lightening Up. What do I need to know at this time?

Inner Guide: Know that you are fine just as you are. That lightening up is simply the process of unburdening yourself of old ways of thinking and doing. Let go of all the things you no longer want or need in your life. Let go of whatever feels like extra baggage. When you feel you're carrying too much, feeling weighed down, stop and let go. Remember, you choose to carry burdens. You choose to let them go. Empty yourself so you can be free to receive the new. Become an open vessel to be filled to overflowing with love.

Drop your fear of not having or being enough. The more you let go of the old, the outworn, the used up parts of your life, the clearer will be your path to the new emerging you. You have my love to guide you.

Thank you, Inner Guide. I will do my best to honor your wisdom and your loving guidance and to realize the truth—that you reside within me.

Yesterday is but a dream, tomorrow is but a vision. But today well lived makes every yesterday a dream of happiness and every tomorrow a vision of hope. Look well, therefore, to this day.

—Indian Proverb

Bibliography

Arenson, Gloria. *How to Stop Playing the Weighting Game*. Granada Hills, CA: Transformation Publications, 1978.

Beattie, Melody. *Codependent No More*. San Francisco: Harper/Hazelden, 1987.

_____. *Beyond Codependency: And Getting Better All the Time*. San Francisco: Harper/Hazelden, 1989.

Borysenko, Ph.D., Joan. *Minding the Body, Mending the Mind*. Reading, MA: Addison-Wesley, 1987.

Capacchione, Lucia, M.A., ATR. *The Creative Journal: The Art of Finding Yourself*. North Hollywood: Newcastle Publishing Co., 1989.

_____. *The Power of Your Other Hand: A Course in Channeling the Inner Wisdom of the Right Brain*. North Hollywood: Newcastle Publishing Co., 1988.

_____. *The Well-Being Journal: Drawing on Your Inner Power to Heal Yourself*. North Hollywood: Newcastle Publishing Co., 1989.

Chernin, Kim. *The Obsession: Reflections on the Tyranny of Slenderness*. New York: Harper & Row, 1981.

Colbin, Annemarie. *Food and Healing: How What You Eat Determines Your Heath, Your Well-Being, and the Quality of Your Life*. New York: Ballantine Books, 1986.

Diamond, Harvey and Marilyn. *Fit For Life*. New York: Warner Books, 1985.

Dychtwald, Ken. *Bodymind*. Los Angeles: J. P. Tarcher, 1977.

Feldenkrais, Moshe. *Awareness Through Movement*. New York: Harper & Row, 1977.

Gawain, Shakti. *Living in the Light*. Mill Valley, CA: Whatever Publishing Inc., 1986.

Hay, Louise. *You Can Heal Your Life*. Santa Monica, CA: Hay House, 1984.

_____. *Love Your Body*. Santa Monica: Hay House, 1989.

Heller, Joseph and Henkin, William A. *Bodywise: Regaining Your Natural Flexibility and Vitality for Maximum Well-Being.* Los Angeles: Jeremy Tarcher, Inc., 1986.

Katzen, Molly. *The Moosewood Cookbook.* Berkeley: Ten Speed Press, 1977.

_____. *Still Life with Menu.* Berkeley, Ten Speed Press, 1988.

Kurtz, Ron and Prestera, Hector, M.D. *The Body Reveals: What Your Body Says About You.* San Francisco: Harper & Row, 1976.

Madison, Deborah with Brown, Edward Espe. *The Greens Cook Book.* New York: Bantam, 1987.

Melody, Pia, with Miller, Andrea Wells, and Miller, J. Keith. *Facing Codependence.* San Francisco: Harper & Row, 1989.

Millman, Marcia. *Such a Pretty Face: Being Fat in America.* New York: W. W. Norton and Company, 1980.

Mindell, Arnold. *Working with the Dreaming Body.* Boston: Routledge & Kegan Paul, 1985.

Orbach, Susie. *Fat is a Feminist Issue.* New York: Paddington Press, 1978.

Pearson, Leonard; Pearson, Lillian; Karola, Saekel. *The Psychologist's Eat Anything Diet.* New York: Popular Library, 1976.

Pierce, Ph.D., Alexandra, and Pierce, Ph.D., Roger. *Expressive Movement: Posture and Action in Daily Life, Sports, and the Performing Arts.* New York: Plenum Press, 1989.

Prudden, Suzy. *MetaFitness: Your Thoughts Taking Shape.* Santa Monica: Hay House, 1989.

Robbins, John. *Diet for a New America: How Your Food Choices Affect Your Health, Happiness, and the Future of Life on Earth.* Walpole, NH: Stillpont Publishing, 1987.

Robertson, Laurel; Flinders, Carol, and Ruppenthal, Brian. *The New Laurel's Kitchen.* Berkeley: Ten Speed Press, 1986.

Rossman, M.D., Martin L. *Healing Yourself: A Step-by-Step Program for Better Health Through Imagery.* New York: Walker and Company, 1987.

Roth, Geneen. *Breaking Free from Compulsive Eating.* New York: The Bobbs-Merrill Company, Inc., 1984.

_____. *Feeding the Hungry Heart.* New York: Signet Book/New American Library, 1983.

Siegel, M.D., Bernie S. *Love, Medicine & Miracles.* New York: Harper & Row, 1986.

_____. *Peace, Love & Healing.* New York: Harper & Row, 1989.

Stone, Christopher. *Re-Creating Your Self.* Portland: Metamorphous Press, Inc. 1988.

Teeguarden, Iona Marsaa. *Acupressure Way of Health.* New York: Japan Publications, 1978.

Vincent, L.M. *Competing with the Sylph: The Pursuit of the Ideal Body Form.* New York: Berkeley Books, 1981.

Whitfield, M.D. Charles L. *Healing the Child Within.* Pompano Beach: Health Communications, 1987.

Williams, Maud Smith. *Growing Straight: The Fitness Secret of the American Indian.* North Hollywood: Newcastle Publishing Co., 1981.

About the Authors

LUCIA CAPACCHIONE, M.A., ATR, is an author, educator, art therapist, and a pioneer in healing through creativity. Originally trained as an artist, she developed her innovative journal method while recovering from a life-threatening illness. She has presented this method in her first two books, *The Creative Journal: The Art of Finding Yourself,* and *The Power of Your Other Hand,* in which she shares her discovery of the therapeutic power of writing and drawing with the non-dominant hand. Lucia has worked extensively with individuals in recovery from addiction and co-dependence, as well as those with cancer, AIDS, and other life-threatening illnesses. She lectures and leads seminars nationwide, trains health-care professionals, and is a creative consultant to corporations. An avid dancer and mother of two grown children, she has authored eight books.

ELIZABETH JOHNSON, M.A., is the author of *As Someone Dies . . . A Handbook for the Living* and co-author (with Lucia Capacchione) of *Lighten Up Journal: Making Friends With Your Body.* As a Creative Journal teacher she developed journal activities for weight loss which she shared with her students and used successfully with herself. She lost thirty pounds in four months without dieting and maintains her ideal weight through journal-keeping and dance classes.

JAMES STROHECKER, B.A., is a writer and creative consultant to publishing. A Phi Beta Kappa graduate of the University of Tennessee with a degree in Anthropology, he has spent the past fifteen years actively exploring systems of transformation and healing. His research has taken him from the excavation of Mayan ruins in Yucatan to three years of study in India. He has edited numerous books on health, healing, and spirituality, including *The Power of Your Other Hand* and *The Picture of Health.* Trained in many body/mind approaches to healing, James has developed *BodyMind Balance,* which integrates deep relaxation, energy awareness and dreamwork with gentle bodywork and movement.